TABLE OF CONTENTS

RATIONAL FASTING

INTRODUCTION 5
I. THE COMMON ROOT CAUSE IN THE NATURE OF ALL DISEASES
. . . . 9
II. MEANS OF ELIMINATING THE COMMON CAUSE OF THE DISEASES AND PREVENTING THEIR RECURRENCE 25
III. THE BASIC CAUSE OF AGING AND UGLINESS, HAIR LOSS AND GRAYING OF THE HAIR 33
IV. DEATH 51
V. APPENDIX. 55

A 49 DAY FASTING EXPERIMENT
PAGE 61

INTRODUCTION

Our modern times have one distinguishing feature in comparison with earlier times: everyone has a different opinion about every question of existence. Not even the scholars, even those of natural science, are unanimous among themselves. They strive to ask more and more questions, to make everything more questionable, until man himself soon becomes a living question mark. Mauthner says in his critique of language a secret that everybody knows: all questions of today are answered with as much "yes" as "no". Of everything that is proved, there is also the counter-proof. This sophistry has even penetrated into science. But the most amazing, the most contradictory, that there can be in human and scientific differences of opinion, is the conception of the nature of the disease. I must no longer hide behind the announcement of my experiences; but I do not have to speak for mankind as such, but for those who want the truth and can bear it, for those who know it from the force of the facts and do not first ask who announces it and whether it does not in the end run counter to the majority of opinions. For more than a year my report in the "Veg. Warte"[1] has been written that I deliberately went with my first student to the malarial region of Italy and that we "waited for the malaria with 45 or 52 pulse beats".

We deliberately slept in the open air in the fever-infested areas and performed the most strenuous marches. I offered to all colonial offices of Europe and America to teach my art of absolute fever resistance to everyone. Today I claim and dare to prove that I am immune to cholera, i.e. that I remain free from it, and that even if I eat unripe fruit, I make everyone immune who lives according to my teachings. It is my duty and moral commandment to publicly proclaim the truth which I have found and which I have tried out on my own body and life, so that it will become obvious to the healthy and they will not sink into the pit of the disease.

---

[1] *Editor note: German magazine Vegetarische Warte.*

There are two main ways for the sick people of today to fight the ailments. The sick want to get over their "sickness" as quickly as possible, to get rid of the pain and the hindrance of the illness as quickly as possible; They have no time to be sick because of all their "work" and probably also because of their inclination for pleasure and enjoyment, and so they resort to pills and mixtures, to serum and tuberculin, to iodine, mercury and Ehrlich Hata[2] and all the other means and remedies, and they really know how to bring about an "improvement" and to keep their heads above water again for a while. But in this way they make a thorough cure more and more impossible and hurry all the more quickly and hopelessly towards the end. Medicine thus simply meets the requirements of time and "downfall". Today's medicine is thus a justified and scientific need of time, to make healthy in the twinkling of an eye, a "scientific miracle," so to speak, and there is no reason to fight it from this point of view. It does full justice to its task, its demand, and is more up to it today than ever before.

The other sick people, they are often called "stupid, backward", in reality they are the honest, intelligent, still viable ones, they want to eliminate the causes of the diseases, which very often are not accepted, they want to pull out the evil by the root, i.e. they want to cure the person, not only to prevent the flames of the disease from burning for hours, days or weeks, and at the same time they want to leave the source of the fire in the body.

Whoever wants to enter this path and make himself healthy again must also be able to take hold of his heart and make sacrifices. He himself is his responsible physician and advisor here; he can only be shown the direction and the path. This is what I make my goal in the current paper.

Between these two extremes lies naturopathy, which gets into an awkward position in that it wants to cure man, but almost always without preventing the disease, the healing process, but also with-

---

[2] *Editor note: Paul Ehrlich (1854–1915) and Sahachiro Hata (1873–1938). Their partnership led to the discovery of arsphenamine, a drug that was introduced at the beginning of the 1910s as the first effective treatment for syphilis, relapsing fever, and African trypanosomiasis. This organoarsenic compound was the first modern antimicrobial agent.*

RATIONAL FASTING

&

A 49 DAY
FASTING EXPERIMENT

ARNOLD EHRET

out eliminating the main cause of the disease, the "good food". To really want to be cured naturally means to live according to the teaching that nature applies in the animal kingdom: fasting and not eating anything "artificial", that is, cooked, that is, only fruit and vegetable. It should not be denied that the individual aids of the natural healing method, the reasonable use of air and water (baths), can still promote the success of the fasting.

How this fasting is to proceed, which foods are to be avoided in general, shall be explained in the following, as far as this is possible, without offending the individual as such and violating the individual healing prescriptions. These prescriptions can only be satisfied by personal advice from case to case. My thinking readers, however, have also derived rich benefit from my previous explanations of a general nature; they will be able to do so all the more definitely from the expanded version.

If the scientific school medicine insists on its medieval exceptional position in the ignoring of an anticipatory layman's discovery, then it judges itself just with it. Has real science, namely natural science and technology, cared whether its discoverers were laymen? However, Franklin and Galvani, Edison and Zeppelin were also mocked, but they respected and acknowledged the penetration of the lay genius. The medical school, however, tells its candidates so casually something about the Priessnitz wrap, but conceals that Priessnitz was a layman.

I do not share the necessarily hostile position against medicine in the camp of naturopathy, nor any current of modern quakery. It must even be shown unequivocally that on this side a boundless charlantery is driven under the "nature" flag. My position and evidence for above assertion is quite exclusive.

I.

THE COMMON ROOT CAUSE
IN THE NATURE OF ALL DISEASES

All phases of the development process of medicine, including those of the first cultural periods, have one thing in common in their conception of the etiological (causal) nature of diseases, that the diseases penetrate into the human being due to external causes and thus, by virtue of a necessary, at least inevitable law, disturb, hurt and finally kill him in his existence. Even modern medicine, as scientifically enlightened as it pretends to be, has not yet escaped this basic demonic conception. Especially the most modern achievement, bacteriology, rejoices over every newly discovered bacillus, as another fellow in the army of beings, which are supposed to be destined to endanger the life of man.

Looking at it in the philosophical light, this conception differs from the medieval superstition and from the age of fetishes[3] only by the exchanged word. Formerly it was an "evil spirit" condensed up to the "satanic character" in the imagination, but now this mischief-making being is a microscopically visible being and its existence is exactly proved.

Admittedly, there is still a big catch with the "disposition". A fine word! But what is to be understood by it, nobody has told us yet. All animal experiments with their symptom reactions do not prove anything for sure, because they only come out when injected into the bloodstream, but never when absorbed into the digestive tract through the mouth.

In the idea of the invasion, in front "coming from outside" of the disease there is something true, even in the case of heredity, but not in the sense that the invader is a spirit (demon) hostile to life or a microscopic being (bacillus), but all diseases without excep-

---

[3] *Editor note: refers to the primitive belief that godly powers can inhere in inanimate things (e.g., in totems)*

tion, even those inherited, come - apart from a few other unhygienic causes - solely from biologically unjust, "unnatural" food and from any kind of disease.

First of all, I maintain that in all diseases, without exception, there is an effort of the organism to excrete mucus[4]) and, in advanced stages, pus (decomposed blood). Every expert will tell me this for all catarrhal symptoms from the harmless cold to the lung inflammation and consumption. Where this secretion of mucus does not openly appear, as in ear, eye, skin and stomach diseases, heart diseases, rheumatism, gout, etc., even in all mental diseases, mucus is nevertheless the main factor of the evil, which is no longer mastered by the natural excretory organs, passes into the blood and produces heat, inflammation, pain, fever at the place in question, where the vascular system is perhaps constricted by too strong a cooling (cold), etc.

If you give a sick person of any kind only "mucusless" food, e.g. fruit or even only water or only lemonade, then the whole digestive energy, which has become free for the first time, throws itself on the mucus masses, which have accumulated since childhood and which have hardened in many cases, as well as on all the "pathological foci"[5] which have arisen from them. And the result? - With absolute certainty, this mucus will appear in the urine and in the feces, which I consider to be the common and main cause of all diseases. If the disease is already in a more advanced stage, so that in some place, even in the deepest interior, there are pathological foci, i.e. decomposed cellular tissue, then pus is also excreted. As soon as the supply of mucus through "artificial food", fatty meat, bread, potatoes, pastries, rice, milk, etc., ceases, the blood stream attacks the mucus and pus of the body itself and discharges it through the urine, in the case of severely infected even through all available openings and the mucous membranes.

If potatoes, grain flour, rice or corresponding meat material is

---

[4] Of course, every healthy organism must also contain a certain amount of mucus, the lymph, a fatty substance of a mucous nature of the intestines, etc.

[5] *Editor note: The main area where an infection starts or a specific part of unhealthy tissue.*

cooked long enough, a gelatinous mucilage or paste is obtained, which is used by bookbinders and carpenters for cardboard and glue. This mucilaginous substance soon becomes acidic, turns into putrefaction, and provides the soil for fungi, molds, and bacilli.

During digestion, which chemically is nothing other than cooking and burning, this mucilage, this paste, is also separated, because the blood can only use the digested glucose that has been converted from starch flour. The excreted, the superfluous metabolic product, this very paste, this mucus, is a foreign substance for the body and is completely excreted in the beginning. Now it must be obvious that in the course of life the intestines and stomach gradually become so agglutinated and slimy that this paste of vegetable origin and this glue of animal origin must turn into putrefaction, clog the blood vessels and finally decompose the stagnant blood. If figs, dates or grapes are cooked thick enough, a paste is also produced, which, however, does not turn into putrefaction and never secretes mucus and which no one calls mucus, but is called syrup. Fructose, the most important for the blood, is also sticky, but is processed by the body as the highest form of fuel and leaves only traces of cellulose for excretion, which, because it is not sticky, is immediately excreted.

Every healthy and sick person deposits stinky mucus on the tongue as soon as he restricts food or fasts. The same happens at the stomach mucosa, of which the tongue is the exact mirror image. This mucus appears during the first defecation after fasting. — Of course, this theory of mucus had to raise dust among those standing on the ground of science, like all discoveries coming from laymen. I must now become even clearer and say what I have not asserted.

I do not say that mucus is always the cause of all diseases, but I say, that it is the common basic factor of all diseases, i.e. there can be many other causes of diseases. I do not deny that there are such, but mucus is always present in every case. It is demonstrably there from childhood even in the supposedly healthy organism. Mucus is in all cases of illness the common and main basis, the main substance in the sum of all disease substances, besides uric acid, metabolic toxins, carbonic acid, etc. It is the residual metabolic products of animal and vegetable origin which, precisely because of their adhesive and glutinous properties, accumulate in the stomach and intestines, become sedentary and gradually clog both. Carried by the bloodstream (white blood cells) into the whole "tube system", especially into the large blood vessels: lungs, heart, kidneys, etc., they cause the clogging of these organs as well. Who refuses to see that a tube about ten meters long, the alimentary canal, gets polluted with time at the inner walls even with the best digestion, cannot be helped.

What I claim is a condition that can be objectively proven by experiment on every human being and not an "amateurish fantasy". I recommend to the doctors and researchers, to verify my assertions by the experiment, which has the sole and only reliable claim to science. The experiment, the question to the nature, is the basis of all natural science and gives the infallible truth, equally valid whether I or another one claims it. Furthermore, I recommend those who are brave enough to verify the experiments described in the following, which I have done on my own body. They will get the same answer from nature, i.e. from their organism, provided that it is healthy in my sense. Up to a certain degree "exactly" the pure, healthy, mucus-less organism reacts. After almost two years of strict fruit diet with intercalated fasting cures, I had reached a degree of health, of which one has no idea nowadays, and which allowed me the following experiments, which I have illuminated in more detail in my work: "A 49-day fasting experiment,", Veg. Warte 1909/10.

I made a knife cut in the forearm; no blood flowed because it immediately thickened; closure of the wound, no inflammation, no pain, no mucus and no pus: healed in three days, blood crust expelled. Later, with vegetarian food including mucilage-formers (starch-flour food), but without eggs and milk: the wound bled a little, hurt and festered slightly, slight inflammation, complete healing only after a longer period. — Later, the same wound with meat food and a little alcohol: prolonged bleeding, the blood bright, red and thin, inflammation, pain, suppuration for several days and healing only after a two-day fasting.

I reported to the Russian War Ministry, in vain, of course, to repeat this experiment. Why did the wounds of the Japanese heal much faster and better in the Russian-Japanese war than those of the "meat and liquor" Russians? For two millennia, no one has ever thought about why the opening of the wrist and even the poison cup could not kill Seneca, after he had previously despised meat and fasted in the dungeon. Seneca is also said to have previously enjoyed only fruit and water. —

All disease is ultimately clogging of the smallest blood vessels, the capillaries, by mucus. No one will want to clean a city's water supply, a system of pipes fed with contaminated water by a pump whose filters are clogged, without stopping the water supply during the cleaning.

No one in the world will want to repair or improve it. Zeder[6] immediately thinks of the control panel, the reservoir and the filters, and these, together with the pumping machine, can only be cleaned as long as the supply is interrupted.

"I am the Lord, the one who heals": only nature heals, cleanses, decongests in the best and infallibly safe way, but only if one stops feeding or at least supply stops. Every "physiological machine", human and animal, immediately cleans itself, dissolves the mucus in the clogged tubes, without standing still, as soon as the supply, at least of solid food, stops. Even in the supposedly healthiest person in Europe, this mucus then appears, as already mentioned above, in the urine, where it can be seen in appropriate jars after it has cooled down. Whoever denies, ignores, or even fights this uniform fact, because it is perhaps too repugnant to him, or not scientific enough, is partly to blame for the undetectability of the main cause of every disease, but this primarily to his own greatest harm. With this, I also uncover the last mystery of pulmonary consumption. Or does anyone believe that this mass of mucus, which a tuberculous person excretes for years, only comes from the lungs themselves? Because these sick people are fed with "mucus" (porridge, milk and fatty meat), there is no end to the mucus until the lungs themselves decay and then the "bacilli" appear and the dissolution is inevitable. The mystery of the bacilli is easy to solve: The accumulation of mucus clogging in the blood vessels over time leads to decomposition, putrefaction of these mucus products

---

[6] *Editor note: The author here most likely mentions Johann Georg Heinrich Zeder, a german zoologist that wrote about visceral worms.*

and dead-cooked food residues These partially decay in the living body (purulent ulcers, cancer, tuberculosis, syphilis, lupus, etc.). Now it is known that meat, cheese and all organic materials in the process of decomposition again "germinate, drive bacilli". Therefore, these germs appear and are detectable only in the higher stage of the disease, but then they are not the cause, but the product of the disease and, however, insofar disease-promoting, as the decomposition, e.g. of the lungs is accelerated by them, because the excretions of the bacilli, their toxins, have a poisoning effect. If it is true that bacilli penetrate from the outside, "infect", then it is only the mucus that enables their activity, gives the suitable soil, the "disposition". As I have already said repeatedly (once every two years) mucus-less, i.e. lived only on fruit. I no longer needed a handkerchief and rarely need this cultural product today. Has one ever seen a healthy animal living in freedom spit or blow its nose? A young physician and naturopath considers my opinion that the nose of a healthy animal or a completely healthy human being should not secrete mucus, nor does it need to secrete mucus, to be erroneous. Meaning a mucus-free nose is pathological. The gentleman seems not to have looked at the nose of an animal in freedom (not a domestic animal). There is absolutely no mucus, but a certain moisture, the precipitation of the water vapor of the cool air with the useful purpose to catch any dust of the inhaled air. If the physician believes that my mucus-free nose is a pathological condition, then I must say that this condition only occurs in quite excellent well-being, when I live completely mucus-free and then it can not possibly be interpreted as a symptom of disease. In the meantime, I have observed the same phenomenon in my patients on a mucus-free diet, and their condition was always the best.

A chronic inflammation of the kidneys, which I had thought to be fatal, was not only cured, but I am now in a state of health and performance that far exceeds that of my healthiest youth. Bring me the European who, at the age of 31, is deathly ill and eight years later can run for nine quarters of an hour and walk for 56 hours.

With this "theory of mucus", confirmed by my repeated experiments, for the first time a thorough, etiological, i.e. the cause designating unity concept of all diseases is established. Even if naturopathy in general speaks here and there of diseases of the blood and Dr. Lahmann in particular speaks of the "dietary blood mixture" as the basic cause of all diseases. This insight has proven to be insufficient, especially in the therapy practiced here, since the dietary regime was designed to be meatless or low in meat, but with bread, porridge, milk, butter, eggs, cheese and flour foods, especially with starch flour foods, all the more mucus was added. This is the reason why most vegetarians are not healthy despite their praised diet. I myself was such a much and mucus eater for several years.

If a larger number of vegetarians do not soon go back to the all-natural diet, the fruit diet, or at least to the mucus-free or mucus-reduced diet, or at least to little eating, then there is a great danger that vegetarianism in its present form will flatten out; not because the principle of "not eating meat" is a bad one, but because the health success with the generally existing vegetarian diet is so inferior. A small number of strict fruit eaters already take the first place in competitions, etc., for which, however, orthodox medicine seeks its explanations elsewhere. The representatives of the vegetarian movement still want to prove what man needs in the way of cooked food, etc., because they themselves do not know what to eat. All the experimenters in this field consider the fruit diet as a remedy that is fundamentally wrong. The hobbyhorse of vegetarian propaganda is to prove that man is not a carnivore and meat is unnatural. The opponents rightly say that eating meat is just as "natural" as eating cabbage, bread, milk and cheese, and so on. Professor v. Bunge accused vegetarians of inconsistency more than a decade ago, and he is right. In the vegetarian scientific camp, under the pressure of the protein theory, the protein and thus the nutritional content of vegetarian food has been measured against that of meat, forgetting the most important principle of all healing, which is: "The more you feed a sick person, the more you harm him" (Hippocrates, an exclusive dietetic, called the greatest physician and father of healing). I am not talking here and until now at all about nutrition in the sense of a way of life, in the sense of vegetarian propaganda, but only about dietetic healing. The mucus-free diet as a healing system conforms to Hippocrates in the sense of not feeding, no longer burdening, eliminating.

Theoretically it is certainly correct that man was formerly a pure fruit eater and biologically correct that he can still be so today. Or perhaps the common sense is not able to see immediately, without any proof, that man, before he became a hunter, lived only on fruits? I even claim: in absolute health, beauty and unimagined power, without pain and suffering, exactly as it is written in the Bible. Only the fruit, the sole "mucus-less" food, is natural. Everything that is prepared or supposedly improved by human hand is evil. The evidence concerning fruit is scientifically accurate; the apple or banana, for example, contains everything that man needs. It is said that there are still old people with great efficiency who have eaten nothing but bananas in their lives. Man is so perfect that he can live on one fruit alone, at least for a long time. But this need not be coconut all the time (Kabakon[7]). But one must not reject a self-evident truth, preached by nature, because nobody could put it into practice for cultural reasons. The well-known coconut apostle Engelhard only made fiasco because he could not cure himself of his tropical disease. Fruit alone will first make you sick, i.e. purified; but it is better to go through the purification process at home and not in the tropics.

No one would have believed me if I had said that in the course of 14 months you could live 126 days, 49 at a time, without food. Now I have done it and people still do not understand this truth. Until now, I only say and teach that fruit is the most natural "remedy". It has nothing to do with nutritional reform here, and whether the Eskimo should and can live like this, whether all people could live like this, why I do not live like this after I was healed. This does not touch the truth of this natural healing system.

Whether my calculation is correct, the next European plague will put it to the test. But I also want to reveal the reasons why people do not believe the self-evident. In the last century, when someone talked about telephoning from Berlin to Paris, people laughed because such a thing had not yet been invented. People no longer believe in natural food, because almost no one can practice it. It is

---

[7] *Editor note: The author mentions the 18-year experiment on Kabakon island by August Engelhardt who lived exclusively on coconuts.*

also important that opponents fear that the prices of other, artificial foods could fall, and others fear that nutritional physiology could be shaken and doctors would become superfluous. Especially the fasting and fruit cures need close supervision and instruction, i.e. more doctors and fewer patients, who, however, are happy to pay more if they become healthy. This would solve the social question of doctors, an assertion I made publicly in Zurich a few years ago.

Almost all fasting attempts fail in ignorance of the fact that, with the exception of the mucus-less diet, old mucus is excreted until the person is completely pure and healthy. This puts the supposedly healthiest person in the state of sickness (purification), in a transit stage to a higher health. Here is the great cliff around which so few vegetarians have so far skirted, which is why they reject the highest truth as much as the masses do. I have proven myself to be competent in this in the "Vegetarian Warte" on the basis of experiments and facts, and with the 49-day fasting experiment with a previous fruit diet I have refuted the greatest objection, that of malnutrition. My condition was only improved by this most radical mucus elimination, apart from some unhygienic circumstances during the experiment. I received numerous acknowledgements, especially from educated people. The general mass of the Vegetarians continue the "mucus". Vegetarianism has representatives of both sexes who have the exact resemblance of the Munich beer bellies; a consequence of the daily stuffing with "mucus food" of the most different kind. On the other hand, the poisons accused by this side: meat, alcohol, coffee and tobacco are relatively harmless in the long run, as long as the same are used moderately. Aren't thousands of people living to a ripe old age, habitual smokers and even often lovers of alcohol? All little eaters — that's the solution! Even these habitual poisons are more innocent than the so-called good and many food.

A drinker can grow old, a glutton never, says Professor Sylvester Graham. In order to prevent misunderstandings on the part of the abstinence movement and vegetarianism, I must insert some clarifications here. Meat is not a food at all, but only a stimulant, which rots in the stomach; the process of rottening does not begin in the stomach, but immediately after slaughter. Graham has already proved this on living humans, and I add to the fact that meat then acts as an irritant and stimulant through the toxins of putrefaction and is thus perceived as a strengthening food. Or can someone prove to me chemico-physiologically that the protein molecule in decomposition is newly transformed in the stomach and celebrates its resurrection, for example, in a muscle of the human being? Just like the alcohol, the meat fakes strength and energy in the beginning, until the whole organism is contaminated with it and the collapse is there. It is similar with the other stimulants.

The basic evil of all non-vegetarian diets is and remains eating too much meat, because it causes all other evils, especially the craving for alcohol. If one eats almost exclusively fruit, the craving for the cup and beer glass falls away by itself, while the meat eater always craves for it, thus has to mortify himself against it, because meat produces the demon thirst. Alcohol is, as it were, a certain antidote for meat and the big city gourmand, who is almost only meat, needs, according to experience, wines, mocha and habana, in order to compensate at least somewhat for the heavy meat poisoning. It is a fact of experience that after an opulent dinner one is mentally and physically much fresher the next day if one makes moderate use of the stimulants, which are poisonous in themselves, than if one stuffs oneself to the point of fatigue with the good food alone. I absolutely declare war on meat and alcohol; by eating fruit and in general already by eating little, the consumption of meat and alcohol is energetically counteracted. But whoever cannot give up meat and alcohol, if he eats very little of it, is decidedly better off than the vegetarian who eats a lot.

The American Fletcher[8] proves this conspicuously by his tremendous successes and his secret is explained by my experiments, which show that man becomes most efficient and develops most perfectly in health, if he eats as little as possible. Aren't the oldest people usually the poorest, thus used to eating little for obvious reasons? Didn't the greatest discoverers and inventors come from

---

[8] *Editor note: The author here mentions Horace Fletcher, a nutritionist whose approach revolved around eating only when hungry, thoroughly chewing the food, and swallowing the chewed food/drinks by sipping (not gulping).*

poor backgrounds, i.e. little eaters? Were not the greatest of mankind, the prophets, founders of religions etc.. ascetics? Is that then culture, that one in Berlin wine and dine finely 3 times a day, and is it social progress that every worker eats 5 times a day and pumps himself full of beer in the evening? The "feast and good food", which until now has been considered harmless, decent, moral and aesthetic, is not only immoral, but more disease-producing than anything else, even among abstainers and vegetarians. If the sick organism can regenerate itself by eating nothing at all, it follows logically that little food is needed for the healthy to remain healthy, strong and enduring.

All the so-called miracles of the saints in the places of grace are only due to spiritual practitioners and are no longer possible today because, although there is much prayer, there is no longer fasting. This is the only solution to this dispute. We have no more miracles because we have no more saints i.e. sanctified and healed by fasting and asceticism (abstinent way of life). The saints were self-luminous, in modern terms mediumistic or spiritual, but only because they were physiologically "divinely" healthy through asceticism and not by "special grace". I want to reveal here only that I myself already made it clear with electric outpourings, but only by external and internal supply of solar energies (sun baths and food from the "sun kitchen", fruit). The whole world is now arguing about these questions and miracles.

Here is the solution based on the experiment that everyone can imitate if he has the courage. But writing books, talking and praying is easier and so is the excuse that I am an exception. That is right, but only as far as courage and knowledge are concerned. Physiologically all people are equal and who cannot moderate himself, he may learn it from me if he wants to be a real researcher. If a man eats little and is healthy, he can digest, i.e. get rid of, the most absurd stuff, meat and starch meal (mucus) for quite some time; he becomes and remains even more perfect and pure, as opposed to if he eats only little fruit, and he needs the least of this, because it is the most perfect food. Today's man does not want to and cannot see this eternal truth of natural law and is justifiably afraid of it, because he is built up of dead-cooked food and his cells fall to death and are eliminated as soon as he sun-bathes, fasts or eats living cells of fruit.

However, this cure must be done with great caution. Medicine has to estimate the human being before the cellular collapse as long as possible, to keep them over water, away from death, but then to let him die of the disease promptly and all the more quickly, which is what is ardently desired today. The vegetarianism cannot deny that the meat and alcohol consumers also have to show a lot of health and great achievements and high age figures but individually and ethnically only as long as little is eaten and not "over-nourished". The too much avenges itself less with meat food, because it contains relatively less "mucus", than with the almost exclusive strong-flour-containing, i.e. "mucusy" vegetarian food and the much-vaunted vegetarian dinners with so and so many courses. I myself have not cared for a meal for many years; I also hurry only when I have an appetite and so little that it does not exert a harmful influence on me if I am also possibly forced to take something that is not in and of itself faultless. The art of staying healthy in today's society is popular less in the what than in the how much of eating and drinking, in the control, in the self-dictated restriction. But to swear oneself to vegetarianism and abstinence, as a pioneer of a hopeless world conversion, and in the end to sin secretly in a sinister mask, I personally consider less exemplary. With this, I would like to thoroughly distance myself from fanatical aspirations.

If fasting can cure the most serious illnesses — this has been proven a thousand times over — and this way of life even makes you stronger, "if you do it right", then the most energetic food, fruit, must make you all the more healthy and strong. This has also been scientifically proven by the deserving physician Dr. Bircher. Although naturopathy has recognized (cf. the term "foreign substances") that something must get out of the sick organism. Up to now it has essentially put the main emphasis on physical stimuli and, as already indicated, it has for the most part completely ignored the really natural moment of the healing process, the reduction of food, the abstention from food and especially the fruit diet, or has only tried to replace it with an alcohol- or meat-free diet. That does not mean much before my "mucus theory". And how do you blame this mucus-free alcohol today. It must now soon be the scapegoat for all diseases, because here and there a reprobate ends up in delirium through immense quantities he consumes. Force a drinker to fast for a few days or to eat only fruit, — I bet that the best bottle will no longer taste good to him. With it one recognizes also that just the whole culture-eating from the Beefsteak up to the allegedly harmless oatmeal the desire for these frowned upon antidotes alcohol, coffee, tea, tobacco produces. Why? Because overeating paralyzes us and stimulants are needed to get us going again. Here lies the true and deepest reason for the increase of alcohol consumption; in the overeating, namely with meat. This is true, because the more acute and stimulating alcohol, especially of modern beer, is in the long run the more harmless than the chronic contamination of the whole digestive tract with mucusy food.

Now I ask: what is more reasonable, to whip out these mucus masses, accumulated since childhood and in decay, which have infected the cellular tissue of the body here and there (symptom of disease), by sweating, bathing, artificial colds (Kneipp cures), massage, sport etc. at the expense of vitality (especially of the heart) and life span from the body or to stop with the supply of mucus? Or does anyone want to prove to me that the best cook or confectioner can make something better, more mucus-free than an apple, grape or banana? If mucus and overeating is the true root cause of all diseases without exception, which I can prove to everyone in his own body, then there can be only one truly natural remedy, i.e. fasting and fruit diet. Even the mucus-free diet may be called a significant step on the way to natural healing. That every animal fasts at the slightest indisposition is well known and proves the correctness of my assertion. Even if our domestic animals, thanks to culture and thanks to the people who feed them, have long since lost their keen instinct for the right food and the natural feeding times - and thus also their health and the sharpness of their senses. In the sick state they take only the most necessary food; they fast themselves healthy. The poor, sick person, on the other hand, must not stay out of mucus food for more than 1-2 days, otherwise he might "lose his strength".

Even doctors have called fasting miracle cures, the cure of the uncured, the cure of all cures, etc. Certain charlatans and self-smart people without any experience have discredited this infallible, but also dangerous cure. I have accomplished in fasting the most significant thing that has been accomplished for centuries: 49 days, world record (see "Vegetarische Warte" 1909 issues 19, 20, 22, 1910 issues 1 and 2). Moreover, I am the first to combine this cure with systematically and individually adapted fruit diet (mucus-free diet), whereby it becomes amazingly easier and absolutely without danger. We are thus demonstrably able to cope with diseases that conventional medicine calls incurable. On the basis of my knowledge that this mucus coming from the cultured food is the basic cause and the main factor in the essence of all diseases, including the symptoms of old age, such as fatness, hair loss, wrinkles, nervous and memory deficiencies, etc.[9]), the justified hope may be expressed regarding the occurrence of a new phase of development of advanced healing methods and biological medicine.

Hippocrates had already recognized the "disease material" for all diseases uniformly. Prof. Dr. Jäger defined the "common reason" as "stench", but did not reveal the source of this "bad smell". Dr. Lahmann and other representatives of the physical-dietary direction, especially Kuhne, were on the trail of these "common substances". But none of them recognized, showed or proved by the experiment that it is this mucus of the cultural food, which from childhood on burdens our whole organism, attacks the latter itself at a certain degree of fermentation, forms pathological foci, i.e. transforms the cellular tissue of the body into pus, into putrefaction. It is activated during an occasional cold or high temperatures, etc., and in an effort to leave the body, causes symptoms of abnormal functions, which until now have been called disease itself.

Thus, it can be said for the first time understandably, what disposition is. The more "mucus" (bad mother's milk and all substitutes) is supplied from childhood or the less as a result of inherited weakness this mucus is excreted by the organs intended for this

---

[9] Aging is a latent disease, see Metchnikow and the latter

purpose, the greater is the tendency (disposition) to catch cold, to fever, to freeze, to cause parasites, to fall ill and to age. Probably with it even the veil of mystery is lifted, which until now still obscures the nature of the white blood cells. I believe that here, as in many other cases, there is an error in medical research. The bacteria attacks the white blood corpuscles, not the other way around, because these consist entirely or largely of this mucus, which is continually accused here. Do you grow bacteria by the millions on this mucus outside the organism? On potato, bouillon, gelatine, i.e. on mucus, i.e. nitrogenous, vegetable or animal substance, consisting of an alkaline reacting liquid, in which granulated cells of the appearance of white blood cells are contained! Perhaps in the completely healthy condition a so-called mucous membrane should not be white, slimy at all, but pure and red, as with an animal. Maybe this "corpse mucus" is even the cause of the paleness of the white rattle? Pale! Corpse color!

With this "mucus theory" to be confirmed by the experiment, the demonic larva of the ghost disease is finally snatched away. Whoever believes me can learn not only to cure himself, even when all else has failed, but for the first time we have been given the means to prevent the disease and make it definitely impossible. Even the dream of perpetual youth and beauty is now is about to become a reality.

The animal organism, especially the human organism, is, mechanically conceived, a complicated tubular system of blood vessels with air gas drive through the lungs, in which the blood fluid is constantly in motion and is regulated by the heart as a valve. The decomposition of the air gas occurs with each breath in the lungs (separation of the air into oxygen and nitrogen; thus the blood is constantly in motion and the human body functions incredibly long without tiring. Completely undiscussed here remains the supersensible, metaphysical concept of a life force, whose existence the purely materialistic way of thinking denies. The thing lies here for us so simply: If we do not break the machine with much food, it runs better!

Don't give me the foolish excuse of the "daily experience of the absolute natural compulsion to eat a lot", which exists for the working man, etc., before you have experienced how easily and how long you can work or march after fasting and on fruit food without getting tired. Tiring is, first, a reduction of strength by too much work of digestion, second, clogging of the heated and consequently constricted blood vessels, and third, "self- and re-poisoning" by the excretion of mucus which takes place during exercise. All organic substances of animal origin, when decomposed, secrete groups of cyanogens, which the chemist Hensel calls bacilli themselves. Air is not only the highest and most perfect operating material of the human body, but also at the same time the first element for construction, repair, replacement, and probably the animal organism absorbs nitrogen also from the air. At least the opposite is not proven. In certain caterpillars an increase in weight by air alone has been observed.

II.

HOW TO ELIMINATE THE COMMON
ROOT CAUSE OF THE DISEASES AND
PREVENT THEIR RECURRENCE

Having taught my readers in the preceding chapter the horror of being and becoming ill, it is fitting that I show them, in summary and as far as this is possible in general terms, ways and means of successfully combating this greatest enemy of health, mucus.
I have already indicated that individual treatment is necessary for the sick person. I have already been able to intervene in numerous and difficult cases in the form of oral and written consultations — the latter only after detailed reports from the patients — to help and heal. Here I would like to show three ways and means that can create change.

1. The shortest and most effective way is fasting, which is much discussed in this book. It makes life miserable for the fierce evildoer in our body, forces him to flee, and with terror he turns away from us, the pheasants.

    Good people can undergo a fasting cure without further ado; of course, they must also fast sensibly and bear the responsibility for it, since they do not cause dangerous overexertion during the folding period by subjecting themselves to physical or mental strain which they would not be able to withstand even on a full diet. One precautionary measure should be mentioned here, which must be applied to all fasting cures: the complete emptying of the bowels at the beginning by a harmless laxative or by an enema, or by both. It is in the nature of things that the person who fasts must not also be troubled by the gases and decomposition substances that form from the feces that remain in the intestines; it is enough that the mucus in its excretion causes the person just enough trouble, which has already been discussed.

    If one doesn't dare to fast for a longer period of time, even though they are healthy, they can do a very short one. Even a 36-hour fast, repeated once or twice a week, has a very beneficial effect over time. The best way to start is to skip the evening meal and take an enema instead. Now, after 36 hours of fasting, one does not eat anything until the next morning and takes only fruits for breakfast. Eating fruits is necessary after each fasting, because the fruit juices make the loosened mucus masses roll; however, in sick and elderly people, this must be carefully individualized. In particular, one-sided meat eaters are urgently warned against immediate fasting and strict fruit diets. This abrupt change can be dangerous. A strictly individualized transition diet under expert guidance and even better supervision is an absolute requirement.

You will reach your goal much faster if you fast for a longer period of time, e.g. three days, and then fasting for several more days. So for three days eat nothing at all, drink only lemonade sips as needed, from the fourth day onwards start with vegetables, salads or fruits and in the evening of the fourth day take an extensive enema. Fasting can be extended to weeks by healthy people and especially by those whose profession allows them to go to their camp during the difficult times of mucus secretions and barometric fluctuations. I always emphasize, however, that these suggestions apply only to relatively healthy people who want to convince themselves by practical experimentation of the spiritual and physical regeneration through fasting. Sick people may not proceed according to such general rules without danger; they must be treated individually. No one should be offended by the so-called bad appearance and the loss of body weight during a fasting attempt. The body fasts itself healthy despite the miserable face color and soon the cheek will decorate a fresh and healthy red and also the weight lifts itself very soon after the fasting again on the normal measure. After fasting, the body reacts to every gram of food. Very moderate and often fasting people have a very fine, spiritualized facial expression. Pope Leo XIII, this great faster and artist of life, is said to have possessed a very clear, almost transparent complexion.

It is worth mentioning in this summary one more point that has already been mentioned elsewhere. The success of fasting depends essentially on it. The fasting person must not be unnecessarily discouraged and must not become a head hanger; for one, rest facilitates the unpleasant moments, for the other, a firm grip when working, especially in light mechanical tasks. Once the body has been de-sludged, de-slimed and de-glutted, it is the sacred duty of the healthy person to hold high the highest earthly happiness he has regained and to preserve it through proper nutrition. About it briefly in the following.

2. Those who cannot fast for health reasons, e.g. because of advanced lung or heart disease, should at least see to it that the accumulation of mucus in the body is stopped by abstaining as much as possible from mucus-forming substances, especially from all flour (cakes), rice and potato dishes, from cooked milk, cheese, meat, etc. The same applies to yogurt. Curd cheese (quark), sour milk, yogurt are less slimy because they also have a draining effect. If you can't do without bread completely, eat black bread and white bread only when toasted; toasting makes it less harmful because the mucilage is partially destroyed. Eating toasted bread also has the advantage that you don't eat so much of it at all, you can't devour it in a predatory manner, and the necessary chewing movements eventually tire the greediest palate.
Those who cannot easily bite toasted bread due to bad teeth may suck on it until the bread has dissolved - an excellent means of raising depleted strength. Those who cannot completely avoid potatoes should only eat them fried. Again, I strongly warn the patient against independent action without expert guidance. Even every small swing to the side of the mucus-free and mucus-poor diet requires modified forms according to illness and individuality. The right and proper transitional diet is very important. It is not decided by the patient, not by his relatives, but only by the expert dietician. Particularly in the case of lung patients, it is often necessary to prevent too severe an attack for months by maintaining a few mucus-forming agents. In this case, my low-mucus prepara-

tions[10] also do a good job.

But what is actually left for me as "strong food", after I should completely avoid the protein-containing meat and enjoy as little as possible of the legumes, e.g. dried peas, lentils, beans? — Some of my readers will ask with a sigh. — I have spoken elsewhere about the value of meat. The small protein requirement can be completely covered by sugary fruits; the banana, the nuts, these in connection with a pair of figs or dates, are muscle builders and strength donors of the first rank. The vegetables (possibly cut into small pieces and processed into salads), the salads themselves, prepared with oil and plenty of lemons, and all the marvelous fruits and berries, those of the south included, are worth covering a gods table. And doesn't Mother Nature come to us in the spring, when our splendid fruits, especially the apples, come to an end and the fresh vegetables have not yet flourished, come to our aid with the glorious oranges from the South?

Will not the fragrance and blessing that emanates from these delicious fruits entice man to gradually become a fruit eater altogether?

It is not possible for me here to go into the diet and its effects in detail; for healthy people this information may suffice, for sick people I will give special instructions at their request, depending on their illness and their particular condition. It should also be mentioned that non-fasters and the slightly ill can and should at least switch on the morning fast. No one would want to eat before noon or at least not before 10 o'clock, and only fruits! The reward of this small mortification is certainly not missing, if it is carried out consistently.

3.   Now a word to those who think they cannot give up the usual mucilaginous food (meat etc.). For them, too, there is a healthy way of eating: "Fletcherizing", i.e. chewing food of any kind according to the method of the American Fletscher

---

[10] Low-mucus vegetable broth, soup for strength, healing aroma, fasting drink, etc. Only available from Mrs. A. Kummer, Biandal-Werk, Köln-Sülz and in the relevant health food stores.

thoroughly, up to liquid mush. At present this method of eating threatens to degenerate in the reform camp and in many cases one must warn against exaggeration, because otherwise the intestine, which is accustomed to ballast, will no longer react. This method is suitable only for such sick people as a transition to fasting, who cannot be helped by abstinence and deprivation of meat, or otherwise in very specific cases of illness. In America they make quite clever cures with little meat and warm water.

Once man has become healthy in my sense, i.e. free of mucus, phlegm and germs, through fasting and a strict diet (fruit-diet), and he sticks to this diet, he will of course no longer need to fast. Then food will become a pleasure for him of which he had no idea before. Only here lies for man the way to happiness, to harmony and to the solution of all questions, especially the social ones, because only through this he becomes free of need and comes closest to the divine. (Socrates).

Can man live permanently on fruit? Of course, one does not need to prove that, the whole universe would be a nonsense; it would have a "biological error", if for every bug the dinner is set, except for humans. Besides, it is scientifically proved that in the apple, in the banana, in the coconut alone already everything is contained what a human being needs. A cow lives its life long only from grass, gives 10 liters of milk daily, pulls the plow and is still eaten at the end. Permanently fat, protein (milk), muscle, strength, warmth is digested only from grass (hay). The highest standing animal, the human being, should be the only one built so clumsy that the organic life could not be preserved with him from the plentiful sun kitchen?

The physiology of nutrition today is still caught in the error that only from fat — fat, from animal protein in the human organism — protein develops etc.. One has the naive, chemico-physiologically quite unscientific idea, from like grows like. A protein molecule of a dead ox muscle, in the process of decomposition and developing corpse poisons, is still exposed to boiling heat in the pan, thus completely "killed". In the stomach it is even more decomposed and should then celebrate resurrection in a new atomic composition as a new muscle molecule in the human being, "start" as they say? Also with the so-called fattening cures one registers the pound-wise weight increase as health increase. One has the idea that with this superfluous stuffing in the shortest time an increased muscle increase is obtained, and the ill ones share this naivety. In reality, the weight gain is by force, a stagnation of the fed fattening food, a burden of the whole body, which can no longer be excreted. Such sick people gradually suffocate in their own, unexcreted food remains (fattened lung patients).

We do not live from what we eat, but from what we digest, what we assimilate. This realization is very advanced, but I must add to it substantially. Our vital functions are intact, healthy, as long as we are able to expel the surplus of food smoothly; and thus one can say: we actually live healthy only for a time, not because we digest well, but because we expel superfluous things well.

The reform camp has not yet shed these basic errors; the vegetable protein preparations have only replaced the inorganic ones of medicine.

I would like to add a word about learning from and within.

The main obstacle, the sore point of fasting and healing diets is the fact that there are people who become sicker, weaker and even die from not eating or from fruit diets, while for many, especially for relatively healthy people, the opposite is the case. Until now it was said in the first case, even short fasting or fruit weakens, and not only that, but that fruit is digested more difficult than cultural food. This fact is undeniable, but its explanation is false and misleading. The weakness does not occur because of the fruit, but by the existing mucus toxins of the sick, which are dissolved too rapidly by the fruit juices or by fasting, carried away into the blood, and as re-intoxication produce the weakness.

The cleansing process must be slowed down by a transitional diet low in mucus, possibly also by small cultural morsels.

But one should not draw from this again the conclusion that culture food is more nutritious, more easily digestible for such individuals than products of the kitchen and cooks.

If an individual is so hereditarily contaminated by lifelong "protein feeding", by descent from a drunkard or for some other reason, that science speaks of cancer, tuberculosis, etc., he will perish from the process of elevation of his purulent mucus even with this most natural cure, but never from fasting or fruit diet.

Here, it must be left to the individual taste and self-responsibility of the individual to either slowly suffocate by continuing to plug or to venture into the unknown with a last try at good luck, the uncertain. Also for the medical doctor there are incurables, otherwise illness would not be in the scope of the divine at all. A completely regenerated organism will expel as completely unusable any food of culture (luxury or occasional cravings, but only nourishment) that is temporarily given as an exception, which proves all the more the necessity and expediency of the natural diet.

III.

THE BASIC CAUSE OF AGING AND UGLINESS, HAIR LOSS AND
GRAYING OF HAIR

THE NATURAL WAY TO PRESERVE YOUTH AND BEAUTY

After the previous general demonstration that mucus is always the basic cause of diseases and aging, it should now be shown in detail and on the different organs, to what extent the mucus of the cultured food hinders the development of beauty in the human body, and produces symptoms of ugliness and aging.

If the lungs and skin were fed only pure pleasure, sun energy, and the stomach and intestines only sun food, i.e. fruit, which is digested almost completely, and only excretes cellulose free of mucus, glue and germs, then it is not understandable why the tubular system of the human body should become defective, why it should slacken, age and finally fail completely. Instead of the living energy cells of the fruit, one consumes "killed food", which is biologically destined for predators, i.e., chemically altered by air oxidation (putrefaction) and by cooking, dead-boiled energy-rich food.

Especially in the heating channel (stomach and intestines), this tubular machine, slag (mucus) accumulates and slowly clogs the channels and filters (glands). Practical experience shows that this sedentary mucus is much more difficult to expel in vegetarian diets with masses of milk, porridge, rice, potatoes, etc. than in moderate meat eaters. The sum of this contamination results in time in chronic defects, causes aging and is the main factor in the nature of any disease. Aging is therefore a latent disease, i.e. slow but increasing malfunction of the life motor.

The chemistry of food provides the most reliable evidence that malformation and decay have their sources essentially in the mineral poverty of cooked cultured foods.

Can inhuman ugliness, lost beauty and symptoms of old age be attributed to improper nutrition? If so, then beauty and rejuvenation therapy boils down to a dietary cure and a corresponding improvement of food. But since beauty, especially human beauty, cannot be defined absolutely, because everyone has a different taste, I can only limit myself to the essential norms of aesthetic requirements. Even if my taste, despite the fact that I have the experience of an expert in the field of the performing arts, is in contradiction with the general and even the modern artist, I must nevertheless consider my present taste to be healthier than ever.

The white color of corpses and sunless culture men is not beautiful after all and comes mainly from the white corpse color of dead-cooked, false food material. What wonderful color a person could have, who feeds on "bleeding" grapes, cherries and oranges and who still sensibly "air and sunbathes", even the moderns of plein air painting have no idea about. Mucus and lack of nutrients means as much as lack of color. Compare the food tables of Prof. König and you will find that mucus-free food, fruits and vegetables are at the top in terms of their content of necessary nutrients, especially lime.[11] The size of a person, i.e. the circumference of fine bones, depends, for example, essentially on the amount of calcium in the food. The Japanese want to increase their race with meat and thus come from the frying pan into the fire. All deformities, bone deformities and especially tooth decay are due to a lack of lime; the lime is precipitated by boiling milk and vegetables. The terrible lack of minerals in cultured food, especially in meat, is partly to blame for the fact that the toothless human race, proclaimed even by doctors, is not a figment of our imagination. Instead of fruit, one wants to replace these substances by organic preparations. The human organism does not assimilate an atom of mineral substance that has not passed into a plant or fruit, i.e. become organic.

The most modern deformity of the human figure, the fat accumulation, has so dulled our aesthetic feeling in this respect that we no longer know the limit of the normal. I do not consider even the bred "muscular man of classical pattern" to be beautiful and authoritative for the ideal type of the Germanic and Aryan race. Weight, standard and especially girth are too large. Any fat is pathological and to this extent unaesthetic. No animal of freedom is padded with fat like so many humans. The cause is only too much food and too much liquid; flabbiness and clogging of the

---

[11] See adjacent table on pages 35-38

whole vascular system are the consequences. Glucose of the fruits and their nutrient salts are the right sources for solid muscle substance, with which one can rebuild a body defatted and degassed by fasting.

THE IMPORTANT FOODS

Composition and nutritional units according to König, Chemistry of Human Food and Commodities (Berlin, 1903)

Food	Water	Nitrogen substance	Fat	Nitrogen-free extracts	Fiber	Fiber Minerals
Meat and meat products without bones						
Beef fat	54,76	18,92	23,65	—	—	1,08
Lean beef	76,47	20,56	1,74	—	—	1,17
Veal fat	72,31	18,88	7,41	0,07	—	1,33
Lean veal	78,84	19,86	0,82	—	—	0,50
Half fat mutton	75,99	17,11	5,77	—	—	1,33
Pork fat	47,40	14,54	37,34	—	—	0,72
Lean pork	72,57	25,25	6,81	—	—	1,10
Goose	40,87	14,21	44,26	—	—	0,66
Pigeon	75,10	22,14	1,00	0,76	—	1,00
Salmon	67,01	19,73	10,74	—	—	1,39
Eel	57,42	12,83	28,37	0,35	—	0,85
Pike	79,84	18,33	0,47	—	—	1,00
Carp	76,97	21,86	1,09	—	—	1,33
Canned Food						
Mettwurst	20,76	39,88	5,10	5,10	—	6,95
Liver sausage	48,70	26,33	6,38	6,38	—	1,12

35

Dairy and dairy products

Cow's milk	87,27	3,39	3,68	4,94	—	0,72
Butter	13,45	0,76	83,70	0,50	—	1,59
Fat cheese	49,79	18,97	25,87	0,83	—	4,54
Skim cheese	43,06	35,59	12,45	4,22	—	4,68
Chicken eggs	73,67	12,55	12,11	0,55	—	1,12

Cereals and legumes

Rice, hulled	13,17	8,13	1,20	75,50	0,88	1,03
Peas	13,80	23,35	1,88	52,65	5,57	2,75
Lentils	12,33	25,94	1,93	52,84	3,92	3,04

Flours, etc.

Fine wheat flour	12,63	10,68	1,13	74,74	0,30	0,52
Coarse wheat flour	12,58	11,60	1,59	73,39	0,92	1,02
Rye flour	12,58	9,62	1,44	73,84	1,35	1,17
Potato flour	17,76	0,88	0,05	80,68	0,06	0,57
Macaroni	11,89	10,88	0,62	75,55	0,42	0,64

Food	Water	Nitrogen substance	Fat	Nitrogen-free extracts	Fiber	Fiber Minerals
Bread, etc.						
Fine wheat bread	33,66	6,81	0,54	57,80	0,31	0,88
Coarse wheat bread	37,27	8,44	0,91	50,99	1,12	1,27
Rye bread	39,70	6,43	0,14	50,44	0,80	1,49
Root Crops						
Potato	74,93	1,99	0,15	20,86	0,98	1,09
Carrot, large	86,77	1,18	0,29	9,06	1,67	1,03
Celery	84,09	1,48	0,39	11,80	1,40	0,84
Leafy vegetables						
Kohlrabi	85,89	2,87	0,21	8,18	1,68	1,17
Onion	86,51	1,60	0,15	10,38	0,71	0,65
Cucumber	95,36	1,09	0,11	2,21	0,78	0,45
French bean	88,75	2,72	0,14	6,60	1,18	0,61
Cauliflower	90,89	2,48	0,34	4,55	0,91	0,83
Winter cabbage (kale)	80,03	3,99	0,90	11,63	1,88	1,57
White cabbage	90,11	1,83	0,18	5,05	1,65	1,18
Spinach	89,24	3,71	0,50	3,61	0,94	2,00
Lettuce	94,33	1,41	0,31	2,19	0,73	1,03
Sauerkraut	91,43	1,25	0,54	3,85	1,31	1,62

Food	Water	Nitrogen substance	Fat	Nitrogen-free extracts	Fiber	Fiber Minerals
Fruit						
Apples	84,37	0,30	—	12,73	1,98	0,42
Pears	85,83	0,35	—	13,09	0,28	0,29
Plums	81,62	0,78	—	16,76	6,42	1,16
Cherries	80,57	1,29	—	13,63	5,77	0,52
Grapes	79,12	1,01	—	16,18	3,03	0,48
Strawberries	86,99	0,59	0,53	7,33	1,56	0,72
Walnut	7,18	16,74	58,47	12,99	2,97	1,65
Sweet Almonds	6,27	21,40	53,16	13,22	3,65	2,30

The fullness of body and face is in alarming increase; it is ugly and certainly pathological. The most strange thing is that this fatness is not only considered beautiful, but as the expression "brimming with health", while daily experience teaches that the lean, youthful type is more resistant in every respect and preferably reaches old age. Already Mantegazza has stated that the lean type is superior to the fat type in strength. Show me a single 80- or 90-year-old with this fullness, which today is praised as beautiful and healthy, and with which one believes to be able to fatten up tuberculosis. How does it make sense that in the poorest countries, where people are "scientifically undernourished", most of the centenarians are to be found?

If the severely obese do not die of heart disease, cerebral apoplexy or dropsy in their prime, a slow emaciation occurs and the need for food diminishes despite all artificial stimulation of the appetite. The skin, especially of the face, which has been excessively tense, becomes crinkly and wrinkled. It has lost its youthful elasticity because of insufficient and unhealthy blood circulation and lack of light and sun. And now one wants to drive away this skin slackness from the outside with ointment and powder! The nobility and beauty of the facial features, the purity and healthy color of the complexion, the clarity and natural size of the eye, the grace of the expression and the color of the lips age and become ugly to the extent that those mucus masses accumulate in the stomach and intestines, which we recognized above as the central depot from which all symptoms of disease and thus also all symptoms of old age are fed. The "beautiful fullness of the cheeks", by which the nose also becomes thickened, is only a mucus congestion, which, as is well known, comes to an outbreak in the case of the common cold.

I now come to the most important and striking symptom of aging, the falling out and graying of the hair, to which I must devote a whole section, because its occurrence usually brings the first and greatest worries and pains about the coming aging, and here science has hitherto been faced with a riddle.

The modern short cut of the male head hair, as well as the frightening earliness of the bald head, have accustomed even an artistically sensitive eye to this appearance in such a way that we are no longer aware of how seriously the aesthetic and harmonious form of man is disturbed by this free and involuntary "hair removal". Man, who is the "crown of creation" not only intellectually, but also as an aesthetic appearance of nature, is robbed of the glorious crown of his head, the hair ornament. "Living skulls" one could call them, these hairless, hard, beardless and expressionless heads of today! Think, for example, the most beautiful woman with a bald head! What man would not turn away in horror?

Or a fashionable tiger of today hewn out in marble! In addition also the mustache angularly and geometrically formed, or also completely trimmed, now still the modern clothes, which distinguishes itself before that of all centuries by the largest bad taste. And we find that beautiful? One must understand the connection in terms of cultural philosophy and cultural history that exists between taste, clothing, architecture and fine art as the formal language of the intellectualism of a cultural period in order to recognize the alarming deformation of man in this direction, who is supposed to be the most perfect and sublime in beauty that nature has produced.I understand very well the external and practical reasons for which today's man has his beard and hair cut back to a minimum length. The unattractiveness and thus the unaesthetic appearance of hair and beard growth has become so general that in the course of time the need for shaving and the use of millimeter machines has set in of its own accord. In our equalizing, all leveling time, one rightly prefers to cut away this scent and, to a certain extent, openness of the inner man, instead of making a living contribution to the proof of the theory of descent through unattractive, disheveled, uneven and chronically inherited pathological hair. Thus the mistreatment of the hair becomes understandable.

The thought suggests itself to us that the ugliness of an organ or a whole organism is synonymous with its inner disease, i.e., nature reveals inner physiological disturbances "diseases" of an organism by disharmony of its forms and colors. The seriously ill and the dead organism are the most extreme form of this phenomenon. I remind doubters of this view, as well as bad and backward observers of nature, of the law of exception to the rule, and in relation to man, of the fact that we no longer have any idea of the ideal beauty and health of man living completely under natural conditions, neither from the point of view of health nor aesthetics. If the pleasure in beauty is a value judgment in the good sense, then the displeasure, the sensation of ugliness, which the objectively existing color and form dissonances of an organism cause in an aesthetically seeing eye, must to a certain degree include the recognition of the pathological. In recognition of the tremendous zeal for research and the enormous progress of today's science, I would like to express here, as an artistic observer of nature by profession, the opinion that today one looks at nature far too much through the microscope instead of with the natural eyes. I repeat and generalize to a certain extent. To the good and aesthetically sensitive observer of nature, the language of form and color of organisms is synonymous with the value judgment of the inner function, the spirit, the sea of the same, if you will. For the general lack of understanding in this direction, the complete lack of artistic education and especially artistic education in the schools of learning must be held responsible. Here we are faced with an enormous gap in modern intellectual development, which will not be closed so quickly by two- or three-week drawing lessons in the Gymnasium. It is an established fact among experts, that in this respect the greatest scholar, e.g. in a gallery, can disgrace himself with a single word in front of any mediocre art student.

After this short digression we come back to our subject. After we have recognized on the one hand haircut as an aesthetic disturbance in the harmonious overall appearance and artistic perfection of the human form, and on the other hand the poor hair growth as the main cause of the unaesthetic, unattractive form of hair and beard, we now have to deal with the chemical composition of the hair substances, the physical properties, but especially with the physiological and biological significance of the hair. If we succeed in gaining a deeper knowledge of the task and significance especially of the human hair in the healthy and diseased body than has been the case up to now, we shall be shown the sure track where the real causes of hair loss are to be sought.

With it the means for the healing of the baldness (Alopecia) are to be found. In Eulenburg's Real Cyclopaedia of All Medicine, page 458, it says: "The cause of this peculiar, universal baldness (alopecia areata) is not yet clear. General states of weakness, anemia (anemia of the blood), local pains, and the like seem to me to be blamed without foundation." Further on page 549: "the presence of fungi has been repeatedly asserted, but never proved as an etiologic (descent) moment." Eulenburg further writes on page 460: "The therapy (medical doctrine) against alopecia areata lacks any positive basis, and insofar as the same is empirical (according to experience), all reliability, it is neither able to shorten the evil, nor to guard against its outbreak at a new place. To be tried are irritating - alcoholic - ethereal liquids, etc." (Hairtonics! The author.)

We see from this that medicine is powerless against this disease of baldness, as cosmetics and hair tonic chemistry have not yet succeeded in actually conjuring up even a single hair. We read about the composition of hair and similar entities in Dr. Anton Reichenow's Encyclopedia of Natural Sciences, Vol. 4, page 188:

"Horn tissue and other epidermoidal formations such as epidermis, hair, nails, hooves, claws, feathers, whalebone, tortoiseshell, etc. consist of fat, fatty acids, lecithin, cholesterol, pigment bodies.

The inorganic salts of the animal organism, among which silica plays a certain role in hair and feathers, and copper also plays a certain role in colored feathers, consist essentially of the albumioid named as the main substance or keratin, a substance which is very rich (silicon 3-8%) in human hair and which otherwise shows a composition similar to that of protein (with a somewhat lower O and higher R content)," etc. "Normal hair is siliceous earth protein," says the chemist Hensel (Jus. Hensel, Das Leben. Page 369). Furthermore, Reichenow, Vol. 3, page 614: "Hair (functional).

The importance of hair is twofold: physiological and biological. The physiological function is a passive protective, warm-keeping layer, in that not only the hairs are poor heat conductors, but also the air, which is held between the hair coat. Furthermore: On the other hand, the cold is a growing stimulus for the hair. The active side of the hairs is their relationship to the sense of touch, etc. The biological meaning lies partly in what has been said above about the protection; a more active activity in this direction has recently been determined first for some insects by Fritz Müller, then generally for all hairy animals by G. Jäger, namely their meaning "as scent organs". F. Müller proved (see Kosmos 1877) that the males of some butterflies possess pads of hair-like scales on certain parts of their bodies, which lie covered when at rest, but when unfolded spread a strong specific scent, the significance of which as a love charm for the opposite sex was correctly recognized by F. Müller. Later, G. Jäger proved that all sharks have the function of scent organs in the following way: "The hair substance especially of mammals has a special absorption capacity for the scents chemically related to musk, which are absolutely peculiar to the respective species, even to the individual individuals, and which are fragrant to the producer and his conspecifics, while they have a much lower absorption capacity for the malodorous exhalations of their carrier. This absorption follows the general laws of absorption, i.e. the lower the temperature, the greater the quantity of scent absorbed, and if the temperature rises, part of this scent is expelled again and escapes into the atmosphere. Therefore, one can speak of the scent of the hair, which spreads a specific atmosphere around every creature (also of the human being, the author) and influences all creatures, which inhale this scent-saturated atmosphere. This scent plays in the relations of the animals to each other a quite extraordinarily important role, namely with the intersexual relations where the partner hair scent is the carrier of the above love spell. Therefore it is explained, that with many creatures, either once for all with the entrance of the puberty, or however each time again with the rutting time, own parts of particularly developed hair emerge, which one has called in the latter case just downright rutting hair. The better known former case is the appearance of the pubic, beard and armpit hair in humans. A girl's proverb says: "A kiss without a beard is like a soup without salt" and therefore the hair plays a leading role in the preparation of sympathetic means.

They can, by the way, be used to create sympathy not only between the two sexes of the same species, but also between the most diverse creatures; thus, in the case of a purchased dog or horse, sympathetic attachment is immediately produced in the new owner if the latter gives the animal a few hairs to swallow, a procedure common among all natural practitioners, which is far from being superstition. For this sympathy-producing love-scent acts not only by inhalation from the atmosphere, into which it escapes, of course. The more intensely the hair is wound, and the more by increase of body heat the scent is driven out of the hair, but also by licking (kissing or swallowing the hair). Further G. Jäger has brought to light the fact, known to primitive peoples and natural practitioners, as well as the physicians of earlier centuries, especially the Paracelsians, but unknown to modern physiology, that this hair scent is not only a general type of nerve, like musk, castoreum, civet, but the specific health substance of the animal, a remedy for its own carrier, of fully specific effect, at least equal — if not superior — to the specific medicines from the plant kingdom. G. Jäger expresses the well-founded assumption that that with which the modern magnetizers accomplish their undeniable healings, and which they call healing or life magnetism, is nothing else than the specific and individual scent in all skin sebum and epidermis formations, not only in hair fat. G. Jäger has introduced the respective scent of man under the name "antrophy" into the healing practice. Furthermore, about the composition and structure of the hair here what Dr. Joh. Ranke writes in his book "The human being" page 160: "The sulfur content of the hair substance is so loosely bound that hair blackens already by contact with metallic lead. The hair cortex is the headquarters of the hair pigment, the hair dye, which occurs both dissolved and in granules and fine distribution."

Page 163: "The life span of the head hair is 2-4 years according to Pinons. It is striking that high-grade baldness is less common in women than in men.[12]) Page 165: "By the investigations of Berthold, hair grows more rapidly by day than by night, more rapidly in the warmer than in the colder season, shaving accelerates the growth of hair, beard hair grows twice as rapidly when shaved every 12 hours as when shaved only every 36 hours." Page 166: "Landois recognized as the next cause of sudden graying the increased air exposure from stretch to stretch." Page 171: "The European peoples are particularly low in this respect, they possess, perhaps as a result of adverse effects of culture, the greatest number of bald and gray heads, and on the average the onset of graying is earliest among them...." What A. V. Humboldt says about this is very characteristic: "Travelers who judge only by the physiognomy of the Indians are tempted to believe that there are few old people among them, and really it is also very difficult to get an idea of the age of the natives unless one can examine the registers of the parishes, which, by the way, are eaten up by the termites every 20-30 years in the hot regions. They themselves, namely the poor Indian country people in New Spain[13], usually never know how old they are. Their hair is never gray, and it is infinitely rarer to find an Indian than a Negro with white hair; moreover, the skin of the Indian does not wrinkle so easily. Often, therefore, one sees in Mexico, in the temperate zone from the Cordilleras, the natives and especially their women reach an age of a hundred years. Such an age is usually fortunate, in that the Mexican and Peruvian Indians preserve their muscular strength until death." Humboldt then

---

[12] Because women generally live more simply than men and do not have their hair cut.

[13] *Editor note: New Spain was an integral territorial entity of the Spanish Empire established during the Spanish conquest of the Americas in 1535.*

mentions an Indian who lived to be 143 years old and walked 3-4 hours a day until he was 130.

About the structure of the human hair of the head, which is microscopically investigated as well as all fibers of the body, without leading a step forward in the elucidation of the concept of the essence of the of the disease (despite the bacilli) to lead a step forward, is briefly mentioned: The hairs are formed by the dermis and consist of medullary and cortical substance and cuticle. The root sits with the hair bulb on the hair papilla, from which growth takes place. Sebaceous glands opening into the hair bellows cause the greasing. The color is caused by dye and by air in the medulla. When graying, the dye winds and increases the air spaces. The growth of the main hair is 0.2 to 0.3 millimeters per day. A human hair carries an average of 180 grams; hair is very hygroscopic (attracts moisture); dry hair becomes electric by rubbing. Falling hairs grow back rapidly as long as the papillae are viable. It has been calculated that the combined length of all hairs cut off during a man's life is 11 to 14 tenants. This fact alone proves how much nature cares for this inconspicuous organ, and yet consider what force and how many good and important substances the body must expend to replace the cut pieces again. I have been thinking about this interesting problem since I was 16 years old. My father was shaved two hours before his death, and on the day of his burial, that is, the third day after, his beard had grown so much again that it would have been easy to shave the dead man once more.

The contraction of skin and muscles due to rigor mortis is not sufficient to explain this strange phenomenon. Similar observations are said to have been made often during excavations of dead bodies, for which, however, I cannot cite any reliable evidence. I would be very grateful for any information in this regard.

For desperate and hopeless bald heads I would like to cite some interesting and scientifically impeccable facts:

Eulenburg, Realencyclopädie der gesamten Heilkunde 1896, Volume I., page 363, says: "According to Albert, a lady lost her blond hair in nervous puerperal fever and it got black, and in another case brown hair was lost after an illness and was replaced by burning red. In the case of a 66-year-old woman, the age-gray hair is said to have turned black shortly before her death. Geigel reports that the blond hair of a lady fell out after severe typhoid fever and black hair grew back in its place."

In agreement with Prof. Dr. Jäger, I have already described above the hair, especially the main human hair, as scent organs of the body, which have to discharge the vapors of the body. Everyone knows that the head and armpits are the first places to sweat, and that sweat, especially in the sick, is associated with a malodorous odor. For this reason, Prof. Dr. Jäger defined illness as "stench" in another place. This seems to me, with exceptions of course, to be correct insofar as I establish the following basic unit concept of disease on the basis of many years of observation and experiments: The disease is caused by the presence of excess mucus and natural food material that has accumulated in the digestive organs over time and appears as mucus secretion.

So, in the deepest and last reason, it is the chemical decay, the decomposition of cell protein. This process is accompanied by stench as is known, while nature connects the emergence of new life with good smell (blooming time of the plants). Actually, the perfectly healthy human being should radiate fragrance and especially his hair. The poets rightly compare the human being with a flower and speak of the hair scent of the woman. So I recognize in the human hair a very important organ, which has, apart from estimating and heat-regulating purposes, the most important and useful function of deriving the exhalations, the scent of the healthy and sick person, which reveals to connoisseurs and good noses not only individual qualities, but even certain information about the inner state of health or illness of a person. If physicians have not yet recognized digestive disorders with a microscope and a test tube, then certain hair doctors have detected the internal putrefaction process that produces stank, the disease, by means of a simple hair diagnosis. Even today, young people who are bursting with health smell like a cesspool coming out of their mouths and are surprised when their hair falls out. Here I have reached the core of my investigation and observation.

First of all, a word about the appearance of hair. It has been established, as mentioned above, that the gray hair is exposed to the air, and I am of the opinion that this "air" probably consists of stinking gases, or at least is mixed with them. I recommend a sensitive chemist to discover the sulfurous acid here, then the disappearance of the hair dye is explained, since sulfur dioxide is known to bleach organic substances.

It now seems to me to be certain, not only theoretically, but especially on the basis of my interesting experiments on my own body, that the main cause of hair fall out can be internal. If through the scent tubes, so to speak "gas chimney of the head", stinking, corrosive and very probably with sulfur dioxide saturated gases must be discharged continuously instead of natural, fragrant fragrances, it should not surprise us if the hair together with its root gradually becomes pale as a corpse, dies and falls out. With this I claim to have recognized the cause of baldness and to have shown the sure way to cure it. The pictures printed in the appendix speak more than whole volumes, and I add that about ten years ago, at the time of my illness of chronic inflammation of the kidneys, combined with a high degree of nervousness, see picture 3, my hair was more gray and fell out. Now, when I was cured of my severe ailment by taking a dietary cure, I saw at the same time the gray hairs diminish and grow to a fullness as shown in Fig. 8.

So if the cause of hair loss is digestive and metabolic disorders, it can only be cured by reducing these factors. I believe that with this fact, which I have tested on my own body through experimentation, even the completely bald heads may finally draw justified hope, after all hair tonics in the world have failed and must fail in spite of all guarantees. The cause is not an external one and cannot be removed from the outside. One must even warn against many hair products, because they contain too sharp, inorganic substances and thus, like many hair dyes, have a harmful effect.

At most, one could speak of a hair-strengthening herbal tonic, to which the nettle preparations belong. The decisive factor seems to me to be that, in addition to the stinging nettle ingredients, there is a happy admixture of fragrant herbs and essential oils and fatty substances, which correspond in their "scent chord" to that of healthy, youthful hair growth. For those whose hair is already falling out and who are already suffering from baldness and would like to regenerate in this direction, I am at your service with advice. There is no such thing as an average diet, and anyone who has understood me will understand that here, too, individualization is necessary. With the influence of my dietetics on digestion and blood formation I can guarantee that the most severe hair loss will be stopped if my advice is followed correctly.

I recommend every thinking researcher to read Prof. Dr. Jäger's "The Discovery of The Soul" at this occasion. It introduces you scientifically into the mysterious world of scents, which, in my opinion, only elucidates the "last things" and especially those of nutrition and the life of the soul and sex. As is well known, beautiful and luxuriant hair is not only a main moment of pleasure and sexual attraction, but it is itself essentially, as I have shown, the organ of revelation of the rising, blossoming life, like the blossom of the plants. Today's almost frightening number of bald heads must be seen as a symptom of the decline in strength of the individual and the decline of the nation. Full, luxuriant hair growth is therefore not only a sign of youthful life and vigor, full, luxuriant hair growth in turn promotes vigor and energy of life. I have provided living proof that rebirth in this respect is possible even in a death row inmate.

All symptoms of old age are therefore latent disease, accumulation of mucus and obstruction by mucus. Anyone who undergoes a thorough cure for any disease by getting rid of dead cells through a mucus-free diet and possibly through fasting, rejuvenates himself at the same time, and anyone who undertakes a rejuvenation cure thus removes the ground from all and any disease. Nobody wants to believe in this possibility. In every encyclopedia there is a scientific opinion that one should die at the most from metabolic disorder, i.e. mucus congestion, so that life should stop without any disease. That would be the normal but unfortunately the exception, the disease, has become the rule today. If someone would live from youth without mucus, even only from fruit, it would be just as sure that he could neither age nor become ill. I have seen people rejuvenated and beautified by a mucus-less diet that they were no longer recognizable. For thousands of years people have been dreaming, writing poetry and painting the fountain of youth and emotionally seeking it in the stars, in suggestion.

What is not spent for remedies against male weakness (impotence), against infertility, of course everything for free. And how easily some could be helped, first of all by correct and nutritious food from the sun kitchen.

We can hardly imagine with what beauty and with what abilities the paradisiacal "godlike" man was endowed, what a wonderfully strong, pure voice he had! The beautification and strengthening of the voice, indeed the recovery of the lost voice, is a quite astounding symptom in my cure, a particularly telling proof of the downright magnificent effect of my system on the total organism of the sick person. I refer here especially to the wonderful success of the cure, which the Kgl. bayer. Kammersänger Heinrich Knote, Munich, underwent under my direction.

The Münchener Zeitung reviews Knote as Tannhäuser in 18.IV. 1911 as follows: "The radical vegetarianism (better said, the "completely mucus-less food", the author) seems to be good for the singer. Bright and wholesome, fresh and youthful, often powerfully overflowing, the beautiful, elastic, technically so exemplarily formed voice sound. A tone, so light, sure and seemingly so effortless, a legato, a breath control, which can only be found with Caruso. And this plump-less German master tenor is much more than a tenor ... "

I will conclude this chapter with a quotation from Goethe's Faust, Part I:

Mephistopheles:
      My friend, now you speak wisely again
      To rejuvenate you, there is also a natural means;
      But it is in another book
      And is a whimsical chapter.

Faust:
      I want to know.

Mephistopheles:
      You've a method here that needs
      No gold, no doctor, no magician:
      Go straight out into the field,
      Start raking and digging,

Keep yourself and your mind
In a very limited circle,
Feed thyself on unmixed food,
Live with the cattle as cattle, and consider not
To manure the field thou reapest thyself;
That is the best means, believe,
To rejuvenate thee to eighty years!

Faust:

I'm not used to it, I can't be bored
To take the spade in my hand.
The narrow life does not suit me at all.

Mephistopheles:

So it's the witch's turn after all!

IV.

THE DEATH.

In the previous chapters I have established the mucus congestion as the most important cause of disease and aging. Likewise, I have demonstrated the possibility of replacement of worn-out cells. In view of the latter fact, it cannot be denied that the complete stoppage of the human engine can be postponed for a long, long time if the body is built up and maintained with living sun food from childhood. In any case, the body nourished in this way has a great advantage over the bad and all-eaters in that its building blocks are much more durable. With the right way of life, the metabolism is significantly lower, as is the strain on the internal organs, especially the heart and the stomach. A mucus-free organism does not have anywhere near the pulse rate of an overeater, even at peak physical performance. Already from this daily reduction of the loss of strength, this constant reduction of the expenditure of operating energy, an advantage in terms of life span can be mathematically calculated and proven. But doesn't the last riddle, death, solve itself under the all clearing up mucus congestion.

In life-threatening injuries and diseases, the brain and heart are the organs whose dysfunction in the last end results in death. It can be said that in most of the diseases, death is caused by the heart disease. However, science has not yet spoken the last word on heart diseases, but it may be said that the blockage of the blood vessels of the heart, consequently the paralysis of the heart muscle and the destruction of the delicate heart nerves by continuous re-intoxication of the blood is the final cause of death in all chronic diseases. Likewise, the blockage of the delicate blood vessels in the brain and their eventual bursting (cerebral apoplexy), as well as any other complete vascular blockage, leads to the cessation of all vital functions. Of course, there are also other secondary circumstances, e.g., lung disease, insufficient air supply, etc.

Science also cites the overgrowth of white blood cells as a cause of death. This disease process is called a specific disease: Leukemia, in my opinion this means: more mucus than blood. Also otherwise

51

still the most different causes of death are indicated: Self-poisons (autotoxins), poisons of metabolic products, poisonous foreign substances, bacilli and their excretions, re-poisoning etc., alcohol and meat poisons, say teetotalers and vegetarians, and yet these two types die until now just as much from diseases and under the same quite seldom painless phenomena as the drinkers and meat eaters.

If by chance the disease cannot be classified under any other heading, the death certificate will say cachexia, which sounds scholarly and means in German: bad nutritional condition, decay. I now ask, what actually is the killing poison? Today's medical research traces the causes of most cachexia back to the bacilli.

Thus, it also suggests a common basic factor of all diseases, aging and death, and certainly a large part of the symptoms and consequences of disease (death) can be attributed to bacilli. My experimental proof that the mucus is the etiological basic and main factor differs from the bacillus theory only in that the mucus is the breeding ground, the precondition, the primary.

The predominance of the white blood cells, i.e., the white dead substance, over the red sugar and iron substance, is fatal for life. Red, colored and sweet, is the sensual emblem of life and love; white, pale, colorless, bitter, is the mark of strength and of the overhandedness of the mucus, of the slow decline of the universe. It is pure mockery, characteristic of our culture, to perceive the presumed pallor, the corpse color of the city dweller as beautiful and healthy. Even art has not remained free of these views (corpse painters).

The death struggle is to be seen only as a last crisis, as the last attempt of the organism to expel mucus — a last struggle of the still living cells against death and their corpses. If the white, the dead cells, the mucus in the blood, gain the upper hand, not only a mechanical blockage in the heart occurs, but a chemical transformation, a decay, a total poisoning, a sudden putrefaction of the whole blood mass, and the machine stops. "God Almighty has pleased", "We bow to the mysterious power of death" — one is content with that.

"Ignorance is the only tragedy of existence. There is no other," says Peter Altensberg in his Prodromos. So also the last, the supreme cause of all illnesses, of aging, at least of unnatural death, is a spiritual one, a lack of knowledge, a sin that one commits unconsciously and for which one is innocently punished, but punished one is, because in nature, as in the civil code, ignorance does not protect punishment. in nature, as in the Civil Code, ignorance does not protect against punishment.

The purpose of these lines is to help fight ignorance, this pitfall for so many poor people, and to spread knowledge that will be a blessing to the individual and the people in body and soul.

V.

APPENDIX

The simple and self-evident is the unbelievable for today's man; he has lost the sense for it and the belief in it because of all knowledge. Art is already in the process of returning to simplicity and thus to true beauty. Let us hope that it will be the same with truth. It, too, is and must be so simple that it is immediately recognized and does not need to be proven, even if the belief in how simply nature solves its problems is missing (Goethe).

For some readers it may be beneficial and valuable to hear some medical opinions and expert judgments about my experiments. First I would like to speak to the reader myself in a series of photographic images. Their compilation gives a vivid account of my physiognomic transformations from my youth on; they show how I have passed through serious illness and been completely restored. Nature wants to regenerate us through the disease process, she wants to bring us to a real rebirth, to a physiological resurrection in the very meaning of the word. If one wants to rejuvenate oneself before one is sick, one must first do this voluntarily through fasting and living food (fruit). Only when everything bad, rotten, worn out is expelled, nature begins to build the new, rejuvenated human being on the still reasonably good cell foundation. It is natural and obvious that the body looks bad and old during the process of cleansing and purification.

What will be done with the large livestock, what will become of the butchers and brewers? Even the baker's trade will be ruined, the whole business world will go out of joint, etc.! These are the oppressive thoughts of the majority of readers.

I ask you to calm down. Such fears are completely unnecessary. Even if an upheaval were to take place in this respect, it would be so slow that no one would suffer in business. Thousands of years would be necessary for such a change. But I myself do not even believe in it. The paradise of mankind will no longer blossom on the planet earth. All state structures of this earth are built on opposites and arose from opposites; they would have to perish in this form if one only wanted to eat fruit and walk naked. And even if a certain penetration of the masses with the principles of a healthy way of life represented by me were to be thought of, the contradictions would still be in such a way that in this economic transformation process production and demand could regulate themselves very slowly. The paradise of mankind remains a utopia. To live under fruit trees and to feed on them outside the "culture" of mankind will be possible only for a few and will be granted only to a few. The lack of understanding, the lack of self-discipline or unbelief provide the opponents of my teaching for a long time for the predominant majority.

Here in this book it is not about this question; we have to do here with the ill man, not with the ill mankind.

But also many a sick person becomes "puzzled" when suddenly the scales fall from his eyes after reading this book. He has usually gone through all stages of allopathic, homeopathic and all shades of the so-called natural healing methods.

At best, he has exchanged alcohol with seltzer and milk, meat with egg and porridge and is not a little surprised that his suffering does not go away despite all this, despite emphatic application. But he is still skeptical, despite the fact that everything I say is so simple, clear, almost self-evident; the whole state of medicine is nonsense? That is especially the monstrous! First to eat oneself ill and then to become healthy by the opposite? To have toiled and toiled for this misery all one's life for nothing? The testimonies of healings of others will not convince many (I could serve with a wagon load), they are too much under the spell of the conventional. Some will make an effort and eat fruit for 8 days, only to come out of the frying pan into the fire and, insisting on their experiences, condemn the whole teaching. But those who have grasped the meaning and true core of my teaching and have the energy to really live by it, will not have to complain about lack of success. They will find that I have not said a word too much, they will no longer be "sick people", they will be and remain

"Healthy people"

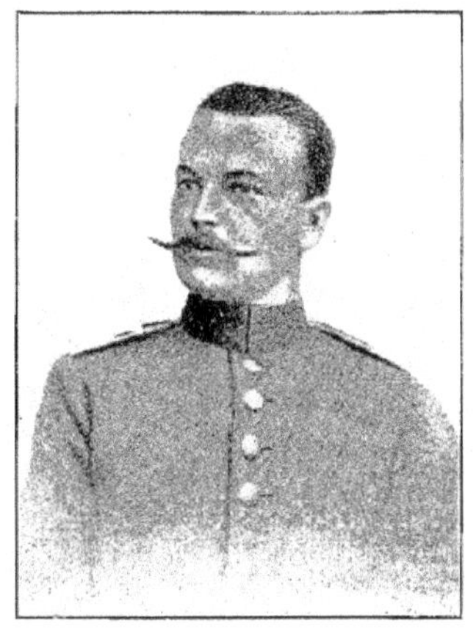

1

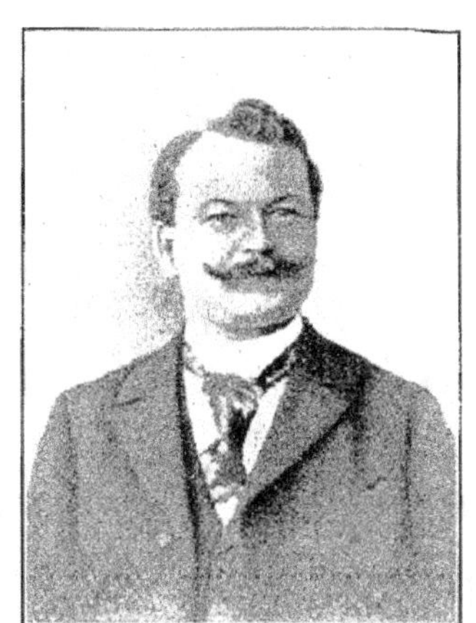

2

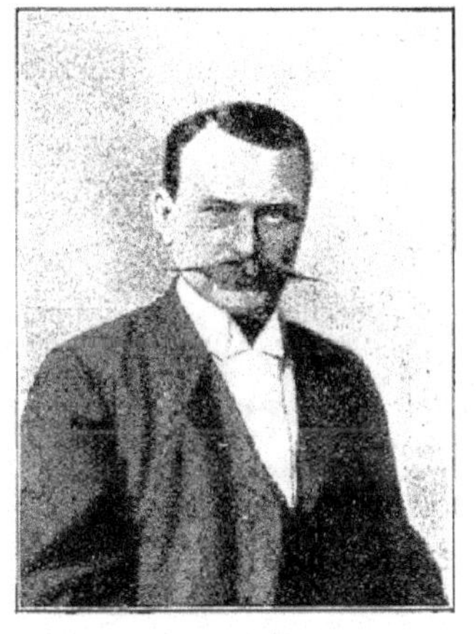

3

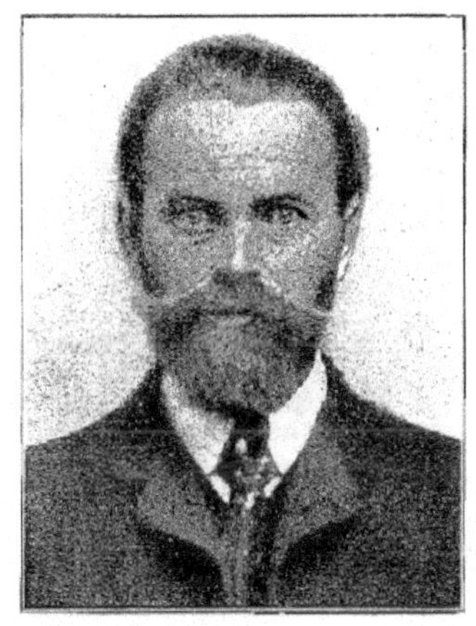

4

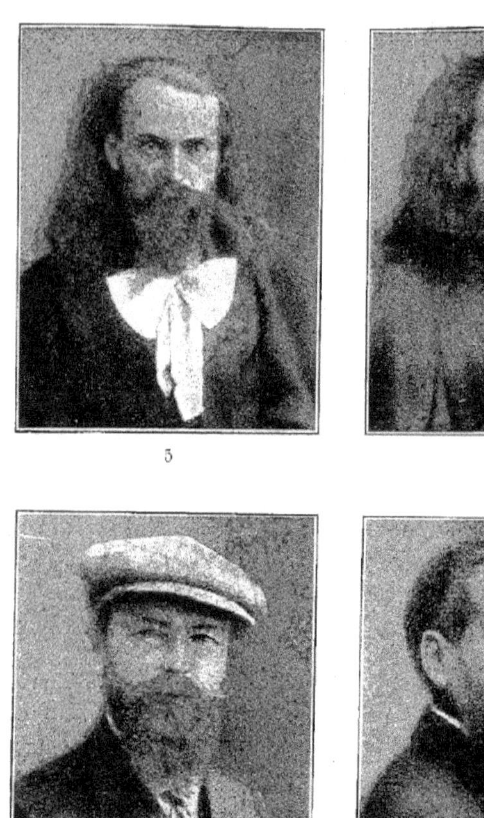

5

6

7

8

Picture 1 is from my military service as a one-year volunteer. Despite my seemingly dashing appearance, I had to be discharged in the 11th month of my service due to neurasthenia and cardiac insufficiency (heart strain). After my recovery and today there are no more traces of cardiac insufficiency.

Picture 2: End of the 20's Shows quite clearly the strain and the intelligence, and mindless expression of today's supposedly healthy frequent eater and beer drinker.

Figure 3: Before the onset of the disease. Already quite a bit of weight loss.

Figure 4: During the disease. Chronic kidney inflammation; father and brother died of lung disease, mother of kidney disease. Approximately two years of allopathic treatment without any success, and close to death. Is estimated to be on average 15 years older than reality.

Figure 5: I was a follower of naturopathy and vegetarianism for several years and found myself much improved, but not completely healthy. At the time this picture was taken, I had returned to a mixed diet, but had already begun fasting. The picture was taken two days after a 32-day fast.

Picture 6: Four days after the same fasting experiment, after two days of eating fruits and feeling unusually strong, lively and mentally alert. At the beginning of my illness, I had suffered from severe hair loss and graying of the hair. The picture shows how my fasting cures also had a regenerating effect on hair growth.

Picture 7 and 8: New pictures after my complete recovery.

A 49-DAY FASTING EXPERIMENT

(Vegetarian Warte 1909: Nr. 19, 20 and 22, 1910)

My fasting experiment of seven weeks, undertaken this summer, is the conclusion of a series of dietary experiments which I have undertaken during the last 12 years, and the important instructive results of which I am herewith submitting to the public for the first time. In fact, my successes have been so much in favor of the vegetarian diet and especially the fruit diet that it is here to be presented to vegetarians. I have degraded myself to an artist by letting myself be locked up in a glass cell sealed by the Royal Notary Dorst in "Kastan's Panoptikum" in Köln and let the public gawk at me day and night. This happened for three important reasons with which I would like to counter the general prejudice against:

1. To protect myself against the temptation to eat solid food.

2. In order to obtain an official one for the fact that I remained without any trace of solid food. Gone are the tents where one could fast as a hermit in the forest and thus find faith.

3. To bring the doctrine of fasting to the general public. Thus, on June 26, 1909, in the evening at 8 o'clock, after I had given a lecture on the effect of fasting on the human body, I was locked up in the cell that had been carefully examined beforehand, and the cell was sealed.

For my occupation I had taken with me books, magazines, writing materials, drawing and painting utensils. Furthermore, I had received 125 liters of Birresborn water, which, however, also had to serve me as washing water. In the cell there was also a good bed, because it is very important to rest well and sleep is more necessary than eating, which I will talk about later. I also had at my disposal: an automatic scale, a portable electric fan and an electric foot warmer. My clothing consisted of a reform suit of my own cut.

My cell was 3m high, had a 30cm high plaster base at the bottom and a 60cm high insert of the finest filigree gauze at the top, which allowed air to enter. Glass panels 1.60m high were inserted between the two. In order to allow correspondence, a gap had been made in one of the strips, which was only formed by a saw cut and was just sufficient to allow a postcard to pass through. The only way to get a letter through was to open it and push the sheets through the gap one by one.

I intended to fast for 51 days, but had to stop after 49 days because I was suffering from very unhealthy conditions. The lack of light and air, but especially the lack of rest and sleep, made this attempt far more difficult than the earlier ones I had carried out in complete freedom.

Fresh air is the first and most important food. If it is abundant, then the loss of strength during fasting is much less.

In the panopticon, I would have risked my life if I had breathed the air produced by the spectators expected in the hall on the last two days. I therefore demanded that the cell be opened after 49 days.

A local newspaper wrote about it: "After 51 active fasts, the liberation of the starving artist Arnold Ehret alias Num Nasor from his notarially sealed glass house in Kastan's Panoptikum was to take place last night. As is well known, things always turn out differently than one thinks. The management of the Panoptikum also had to learn this. In fact, the "man who knows sheep" (Arabic: Num Nasar) was supposed to be the one who gave them sleepless nights. However, the ability to sleep expressed in the name "Num Nasar" had only theoretical meaning in the last time, because in practice the unseemly behavior of many nocturnal visitors disturbed the slumber of Num Nasar so necessary for the realization of the experiment for quite a while. And to this circumstance it will be to be attributed probably in the first place if the fasting artist did not reach the set goal completely. Last Saturday, alarming disturbances in his well-being took on a threatening character, so that the management, in its sense of responsibility, felt compelled to have a doctor come and, after notarially unsealing Num Nasar's cell, to have him examine him. The doctor's advice was to end the fasting, which had already lasted 49 days, as soon as possible. However, Num Nazar's tenacious willpower initially refused to comply with the instruction and demanded that the experiment be continued until its programmed end. However, the cell had hardly been sealed again by the notary when nervous crises set in again, which defeated even the energy of Num Nazar. (Result of the mass visitation of the last days. A.E.) So he was released two days before the planned date. But the lack of 48 hours does not diminish the astonishment that a feat of fasting like that of Arnold Ehret, who was able to abstain from any food for 49 days, demands from us".

You can see from this that my energy had still not left me. But everything has its limits.

With 49 days, I had set a new, unmatched world record in fasting. Because the famous professional hunger artist Ricardo Sacco calls himself world champion of hunger art due to an experiment of 47 days in Wroclaw. He now wants to fast for 55 days to beat me. He may calm down his worry about my competition, because I do not perform the fasting professionally, but for purely scientific reasons and also conclude with this publicly great experiments.

Although the Panoptikum had sent circulars to the medical profession of Köln with some medical reports, which clarified the reliability and the reality as well as the scientific value of my experiments, only one (Dr. M.) had taken an open interest in it. However, his orders became fatal for me in that they cut off the possibility of maintaining my diet (drinks and food), which had already been tested many times, after the fasting experiment. The consequence of this is that at the time of writing this essay I am still not quite up on my feet, while otherwise I was already awake the other day, even after 32 days of fasting. I will come back to the diet after fasting as a remedy in more detail in the second part, the theoretical part. I only want to note that the most important and dangerous moment of the whole experiment lies here and that all dilettantism in fasting cures must be firmly warned against. If exact instructions are not given by an experienced physician or other good practitioner supervising the cure, depending on the illness, number of fasting days, individuality, time of year, etc., there is a danger to life, especially if in fear stimulants such as coffee beans, alcohol, bouillon, etc. are resorted to.

Usually around the time of the 11th to the 13th day, the so-called critical time, certain states of weakness set in, which, if they are increased by death angst of the inexperienced and the independently proceeding dilettante, can become alarming. But the condition increases with time, it does not even last, and thus under certain circumstances one can be more efficient again on the 17th or 18th day than on the thirteenth. In Köln, for example, I was able to lift a weight of 30 pounds more often on the 17th day than a few days before. Up to a certain point, the decrease in strength does not progress with the number of fasting days, but rather in a curve. From about the 40th day, however, a persistent state of weakness occurred in Köln. I believe, however, that in fresh, dust-free air and with sufficient rest, strength is preserved far longer. In Köln, although I have achieved a certain sleep art through auto-suggestion similar to that of the fakirs, I was not able to sleep quietly for half an hour during the entire 49 days, since the Panoptikum was open day and night without interruption, at the same time for the control of reality by the audience. But even the employed staff was as inconsiderate in their noisy entertainment as the often drunken night visitors, despite my repeated requests. On the so-called critical days, the great mental strain is to be emphasized, which, however, brings with it the danger for the beginner that he will not overcome the temptation to eat in his anxiety and mood, if he does not have an experienced practitioner at his side, who can morally straighten him out. For the mental moment plays a greater role in a fasting cure, especially in a sick person, than in any other. Therefore, this cure must be managed and supervised more carefully than any other. In fact, only a few patients should be treated under constant supervision. But then the success is so much more certain.

My weight decreased by 41 pounds during these days, much of which was due to insomnia. I drank an average of 1/2 liters of water daily. In addition to mineral water, I also took some laxative tea and a few peppermint tablets against thirst and coughing, which, by the way, do not count as food. I hardly used them. So I lived 49 days with about 60 liters of mineral water under unhygienic conditions and with sleeplessness caused by disturbance. The pulse and heart activity remained normal until the last day. Within a period of one year I have fasted for a total of 105 days and I dare to say that on average I have overfed and that this unique experiment has not only not harmed my health, but even benefited it. I have been a vegetarian for 6 years. For about 2 years I lived strictly on fruit, even in the cold winter!

From time to time, partly on purpose for experimental purposes, partly out of indifference, I ate some meat, but then also some wine or beer with the meat. For weeks before the great fast I lived strictly vegetarian, almost only on fruit; only coffee and the cigar I did not completely Hess. However, to counter the prejudices in this regard, I will note that I survived an earlier rather extended fasting attempt more easily without any significant loss of strength because I had eaten essentially only cherries four weeks earlier. This experimental fact may sound almost insane even to the ears of the radical vegetarian, and even more so to those of the meat eater and orthodox physician. But it remains therefore nevertheless as a fact and proves evenly more than thousand volumes that in relation to metabolism, nutrition, illness concept, fasting and the abilities of the perfectly healthy person generally the last truth is still far not fathomed. In my further explanations, I will set up completely new, partly unheard-of views based on the facts of experience and, above all, I will try to prove that fasting is not only the best, safest and, above all, the most natural remedy, but that here is a highly important contribution to the solution of the whole mystery of mankind, yes, even that here is the most interesting problem that there can be for the whole of mankind. The philosopher of the "revaluation of all values", Friedrich Nietzsche, said in one place of his works: "I pride myself to say in one sentence what another needs volumes for". Another saying of his is, at least according to the sense: "A so-called truth, which must first be proved, is in itself doubtful." I will now set forth two propositions which alone contain the whole epitome of all knowledge, are the alpha and omega of all wisdom, because the one, if correct, reveals the root cause of all evil in the world, and the other at least gives the key to the solution of all questions and riddles and the means by which the human can be raised to a paradisiacal perfection in physical and spiritual relation.

To both of these theses also Nietzsche's word applies that it should actually need no proof to recognize the nature and the composition of the human blood and the place of its preparation, the alimentary canal, as the starting point, the deciding factor, the determining factor in the whole physical and spiritual life of man. This is actually as self-evident as any truth, namely also as far as the mental and spiritual functions, the way of thinking and the world view itself are concerned. Not only the structure and form of the brain is decisive for the mental and spiritual abilities, but rather the nature of the blood, by which the brain is nourished. Since nowadays the most learned and "spiritually rich" are blind to the simple things of life, this can also be proved to them, because they have lost all faith. Their distrust against the life and the nature and with it their whole pessimism goes so far that they, for example mentioned, do not even admit that no cook and no confectioner of the world can bring about something more perfect than an apple or banana!

Still I would like to avoid the suspicion, as if I represent a one-sided crass materialism. I am even a decided supporter of the primacy of the spirit before the matter, what I also believe to have proved by my great fasting experiment. Here it is a question of the influence of such material effects on soul and spirit, as they have not yet been set forth clearly enough. My two content-heavy sentences are:

1. All sickness, pain, sorrow and suffering, all passions, alcoholism (even morphine and tobacco consumption), all "evil," the whole social struggle, the inequality of men, overpopulation, war, cruelty, slavery and servitude (also that of woman by the kitchen), human deformity, aging and perhaps even death itself, all philosophical and moral heresies, but especially pessimism, in short all degeneracy, comes, except in a few circumstances, from wrong, unnatural food and from overeating.

2. Fasting is the only means applied by nature without human intervention to repair the consequences of overeating, even the "sins of the fathers", and if combined with the pure natural diet (strict fruit diet) according to plan, the only infallible way in which all evils could be eliminated from the world!

Theoretically, this is certainly correct according to my experience. However, even I do not believe that mankind could be saved by this, since only a few have the energy to endure this transitory process (disease) demanded by nature, which has been thoroughly misunderstood until now. Before I now go into this in more detail, first my experimental material is to be presented together with some other facts, by which our previous concepts of illness, nutrition, metabolism, sleep, physical and mental abilities of man are put into a different light.

At the age of 30, I collapsed under the burden and work and the consequences of chronic kidney inflammation. I had taught almost twice as many students in a high school as my colleagues, and in addition I had given a lot of private lessons. My mother had died of kidney disease, and my father and brother had died several years earlier of consumption of the lungs. At the age of 18, I also had an alarming lung catarrh. After I had sought help from a number of doctors and authorities in vain and had already sacrificed a fortune, solely as a result of the increased over-nutrition, I turned to naturopathy and vegetarianism. This improved my condition, and I at least realized that complete healing could only be sought in this direction, even though I was far from being healthy. During a winter stay in Algiers I tried a fruit diet, but I did not get much further, because I did not fast, ate too much and did not know the right selection and composition. Such mistakes are also the main reasons why the representatives of the only correct and strictly natural vegetarianism, the fruit diet, are so in the minority. I will therefore hold theoretical and practical courses, especially here in Locarno, in order to train a certain staff that will be less likely than before - I guarantee it - to fall prey to the ridicule of our opponents.

I began in Algiers with small fasting experiments, but I suffered terribly from the great cliff, the so-called crisis, which is insurmountable for most people, because I still had the idea that the weakness came from the lack of food, while my great experiments and the subsequent achievements prove the opposite. This was the biggest and most fatal mistake in thinking until now.

One day, thanks to my energy, I overcame the crisis, under which I imagined nothing clear just then, and despite great hunger, great weakness and disgruntlement, I sat on the bike until suicide.

Here, to want to overcome matter by spirit and soul means first of all to "believe", i.e. to have confidence in nature and in life, or in other words, if one wants to recognize the physiological sense in the biblical words: "God does not want the death of the sinner (transgression of the laws of nature), but that he should live"! After only half an hour's ride, I noticed that hunger, weakness, and disgruntlement diminished the longer and faster I drove. When I arrived in the town of Blida (48km away), I felt as if reborn, lively, strong, cheerful, and the strangest thing was that hunger had also disappeared completely. I only quenched my thirst with some tangerines, which grow splendidly in this country. But with the realization of this fact, this actually involuntary experiment, the first subversive thoughts against the principles of our diet in general rose in my mind. Two months later, with a trained sportsman, I cycled from Algiers to Biskra and Tunis (about 1000km) in not quite 14 days. Consider: a former death row inmate! Returned to the service, I was forced by the circumstances to eat again "well". After all, today it is a thousand times more difficult to keep from eating sick than to get enough food. I became ill again. Now, together with a young friend, Mr. B., who has remained my most loyal student and follower ever since, I decided to go on a decisive cure and death at my own risk, and to do so far away, namely to escape the "good" advice of the relatives. Which of the many cures and remedies offered even in our camp should be trusted? After fasting for seven days and eating once, we carried our suitcases to the train (in La Eroir, southern France) by ourselves for 1% hours, which would have been impossible for both of us before. After a nine-day fast and two meals (making the right choice in this is the most important thing), we began a march from Nice over the Col di Tenda to Milan. We both felt so lively and strong, and as night fell, the desire to march and the joyful mood increased to such a fabulous degree that we firmly believed that a mysterious power had poured over us. I had never felt such a sense of indefatigable power in my healthiest youth, and in this I never lagged behind my friend who was 12 years younger. I could hardly believe myself now that I had been terminally ill before and had been considered incurable. We had not had any food since Nice. Only at night after 11 o'clock we quenched our thirst in a tavern in the mountains with a lemonade. Neither of us was hungry. So we continued our march at the best pace all night, the other day and the following night, resting only briefly and a few times, taking some fruit or lemonade. Only when we passed through a road tunnel at midnight did we sleep on a bench for barely half an hour, and that was enough to strengthen us both again to such an extent that we were now all the more anxious to make the whole march a test of our almost unearthly strength and to hold out until a pronounced feeling of tiredness set in. However, this had not yet become noticeable by the 56th hour of the march, when a downpour surprised us and we therefore had to use the railroad to reach our destination, the city of Milan. From Milan we walked again to Genoa, without going to an inn, sleeping in the open air. Our strength and full sense of health increased to unimaginable levels on a pure fruit diet. In Genoa we had to wait several days for our luggage, and this big city, where of course we had to stay in the inn, seduced us again to the so-called "good food". With that, however, the cheerful mood and the strength, especially in me, diminished again to the point of morbid discomfort. Doubts about everything set in again. We went to Capri and there I decided to make my most memorable fasting attempt on life and death. Now I wanted to be certain under all circumstances where the truth lay. I would rather perish than remain in this doubt of the uncertain and halfway, where I was never quite healthy and also not quite sick. This is a typical condition of so many followers of naturopathy and vegetarianism, who, if I am not mistaken, are usually called cure hunters. My friend fasted on Capri in a lonely villa for 13 days, by which, with the help of some other order given by me and appropriate diet, he was permanently cured of hitherto incurable stuttering and inherited nervousness. I endured 21 days, being in an indescribable miserable condition for the last 8 days, for which, however, I was soon to be rewarded. After 3 days of food intake, I was finally not only freed from my kidney ailment, but I have since exhibited such a series of outstanding physical and mental achievements as I had never dreamed of in the best full strength of the twenties. I thus not only regained full health, but also my appearance has rejuvenated, as I detailed in my pamphlet on hair diseases, which is now included in my book "Sick People". We marched through the whole of southern Italy, and I underwent a punishing Oriental journey via Brindisi, Egypt, Palestine, Constantinople, Hungary, Vienna and Munich, whereby, to mention this in passing, I used only 1800 marks in 14 months and yet saw everything interesting on my journey. Briefly, the following samples and facts are given to support my views on fasting and fruit diet.

With exclusive grape diet without bread I did 150 squats and poor fruit diet (cherries) and did not do badly without practice. For a number of years I made dietary experiments with great sacrifices and efforts and inconveniences, such as have perhaps not been carried out in this way before, and through which I came to completely different views about many things, such as alcohol, vegetarianism, coffee, etc.. But the most important and decisive thing remained for me the fruit diet and fasting. In Switzerland I underwent two public fasting experiments of 20 and 24 days, and in northern Germany one of 32 days with tap (i.e., not mineral) water, which no one had ever done before. The Köln attempt followed already 2 months later. On the basis of this forward stretching, after seven days of fasting with intake of very small amounts of fruit (a few bites daily) an air bath in nightly snow flurries, combined with 250 knee bends and forward stretching of arms. With an equally small intake of fruit for 11 days, I performed an endurance run of 2 hours in an air bath in the June heat over noon in front of many spectators, including a doctor.. The doctor noted an increase in pulse rate of only 9 beats, while I used to suffer from major heart problems. This also corrects a great error of physiology, which consists in a misunderstanding about the connection between blood and heart, which plays a great role in fasting. As a soldier I was one of the worst shooters due to nervousness (I was discharged in the 11 months of service because of neurasthenia and nervousness). However, after a fasting of 7 days and a two-day fruit diet, I shot so confidently at needles, even moving ones, in a booth at the port in Marseilles with fever without prior practice that the owner commented to me: Monsieur, je n'ai jamais vu comme ca" (I have not seen anything like that). I fasted only with water during heavy agricultural work for 3 days and tired less than the others. I often helped to perform the heaviest work of this kind, namely the mowing, with pure and completely experimental material. I will now illuminate the two preceding theses in more detail in the following. Before I go into the exposition of my peculiar standpoint and my partly new views, I would like to remind you of a number of facts which should make every thinking person waver in our previous conception of nutrition, etc. Professor Graham asserts in his "Physiology of Nutrition" that Kaspar Hauser grew up on water and bread.

Where did he get the nitrogen and lime for his bones? It is scientifically certain that fakirs can be buried for months and live again without being fat, like an animal in hibernation. Where is the metabolism here? The Catholic Church has saints of whom it is proved to the evidence that they have enjoyed almost nothing for years except water and the host, what one can call a perfect fasting according to today's terms. In most cases they even lived to a very old age, and many of them have no less mental or physical achievements to show. In the aquarium in Paris a wildly captured snake remained alive for 3 years without food, and the zoologist Professor Weissmann is said to have observed that a beetle lived for 6 years only with air access, even without water, until it perished. Where is then here the metabolism, which is to receive alone the life? And the human being, "the crown of creation", can hardly skip a meal because of all the assembly and disassembly. I remind of the old man with the earthquake in Messina who lived 28 days only from grass! Now I need to take a position on important, seemingly scientifically established concepts and views, even in the field of natural medicine, in order to then be able to go into more detail on my two theses. The illness, the best-meant physiological process of the nature, in order to let the human being get through to the health, to bring the food remainders and the tissues and muscle cells rotten by diluted blood to the excretion, stands today again in the sign of a pessimistic and demonic conception, and this thanks to the scientifically "enlightened" of the 20th century, who boast to be without superstition, although they fear a single bacillus more than one feared formerly the devil himself. In this sense, there is only one disease.

Even cancer, all ulcers and rash diseases, etc. are, in a sense, only emergency valves, These are nature's means of collecting and transporting outwardly deposited morbid substances and thus protecting the sick person from death. All glandular swellings, thickenings, etc., are temporary deposits to keep the blood as pure as possible, despite the continuous supply of far too much food. Just imagine this mixed food in the stomach of a human being after an abundant feast: soup, meat, pastries, rice, bread, milk, etc., at least five or six times a day, more than would actually be necessary, and, as a result of the continuous drinking, swimming in enormous amounts of liquid! One is surprised when so much mucus is secreted (lung patients), and when finally everything becomes putrid and festering.

The water, an element of the living, in excess becomes the doom of plant, animal and man.

In relation to plants and animals, every farmer knows this, but in relation to humans, the abstainers seem to have forgotten it. I consider wine and beer in modest limits to be good in cases of overeating, precisely because alcohol counteracts protein and fat absorption. The lavish eater does not instinctively reach for this "antidote" for nothing, and Graham already says:

"A drunkard can grow old, a glutton never". That alcohol acts as an "antidote" when eating meat is true. All the more reason for the abstainer to give up eating meat.

Because the vegetarian does not need the "antidote". The nature tries to compensate the overfeeding and the supply of wrong food components with all reserve forces continuously. If it does not succeed any more, it gives a signal, called pain, accompanied by disgruntlement, loss of appetite, fever, etc., which, for example, in the case of toothache, means: "Thou shalt not eat". Instead of obeying, one responds by numbing and tearing out. Because today's people, whose time is filled only by business and pleasure, have no time to be sick, i.e. to become healthier. Today's allopathy and surgery is tailored precisely to this humanity. With all its poisons and serum preparations it merely corresponds to the actual demand and the need of the masses, the "too many". The drugs suppress the warning signal and the symptoms of the healing process (disease) until the last reserve forces are exhausted and death occurs. When one correctly grasps the spirit of illness, one must say: We cannot become ill early enough. Fasting is actually an artificial disease, Only when the filling up stops, the organism gains strength and time to approach the undisturbed excretion of the waste, the "foreign substances" with concentrated blood. If "exhaustion" occurs soon, it does not come from a lack of food, as most vegetarians believe, but solely from self-poisoning. The result is a reduction in the blood count due to the dissolved putrefactive substances, which then leave the body with a terrible stench, if the correct procedure is followed. As soon as this has happened, a greater feeling of strength appears immediately, even without food intake.

But the weakness, called crisis, under which until now nothing proper was imagined, has become all the more fatal for most vegetarians, because they eliminate the stimulants, which just all, including meat allopathic, i.e. in this sense and to some extent "disease-preventing" (i.e. eliminating the crisis). But the vegetarian, who is not a pure fruit eater and usually eats too much, goes only half way. As a result, there is a continuous elimination process in the body, and periodic states of weakness occur, which are mistakenly interpreted as malnutrition. The crises do not cease, and perfect health is never attained. To have clarified this most fatal error by the living attempt and to have refuted it finally, this I count as my merit. Even if similar theories have already existed here and there, it is and remains incompatible with my view if one wants to find malnutrition in me who has set the world record in fasting. So much about the spirit of the disease.

The need for regular meals is perhaps only a disease of the cultured man, because thereby only dead-cooked material is supplied to him; hence the rapid decay. I fundamentally attack the nitrogen theory and no longer believe that a protein molecule in the process of decomposition (skin gout!), which in addition is fried in the boiling heat, celebrates its "resurrection" as a part of the muscle substance of man. Meat and its effect is to be regarded only as stimulant. It seems to me certain that the living substance takes the nitrogen it needs from the air, and that the full-grown healthy man hardly needs any substitute, but almost only operating material. Or should it be a coincidence that the life-conditioning breathing air contains 75 percent nitrogen? Should about the muscle protein of an ox living in freedom come only from the grass? Has that ever been calculated? But where are the "heat calories "*" of a deer at 20 degrees cold. Should the functions of an animal organism be calculable at all? This is the progress of our culture, when every professor tells us something different about what and how much we should eat, and that the "wittiest" scholars and artists believe in things that the stupidest of the darkest Middle Ages would have rejected. This includes, for example, the belief that one could supplement and improve one's daily diet with stinking half-rotten ox blood (hematogen). In general, the whole physiology is based on blatant errors, because the first scholars who founded this science had no thorough knowledge of natural science. For example, they teach that the heart is a pump and causes the circulation of the blood, which in my opinion is the greatest physiological error, which even today most naturopathic physicians still follow. I think that the animal organism can be compared to a gas engine, where the air and its oxygen, through the lungs, pneumatically and chemically (absorbing oxygen) set the blood in motion. The heart is the valve, the regulator of this pumping system. Where should the driving force in the heart come from, if it were different? It could be explained only metaphysically, and one does not believe in such any more today. Does not rather the "course" of the heart depend on the supply of the air as well as on heating and cooling influences? Does not the heart stop as soon as the air ceases to enter the lungs? And the heart is supposed to be the cause of the movement of the blood! However, the heart still performs a few beats when breathing stops, but only until the stimulus exerted by the breathing air ceases and the pneumatic pressure is equalized.

For the first-mentioned reason, a rabbit heart that has been cut out and impaled can be set in motion again after several hours by saline solution or diluted glucose. The scientific misconception about the purpose of the heart, however, is the main culprit in the still mysterious darkness that hovers over all diseases, especially heart diseases. I insist that it is also internal gases, at least odoriferous substances, which support the operation of the heart and sustain life. The odoriferous substances are the carriers of life, which Professor Jäger called soul substances, only with the difference that they stink in humans, because they come from decomposed organic substances of food. The fruit eater, however, apart from the perhaps still necessary substitution, keeps his organism in motion by fragrant odors of the fruit. These are the real and proper energies which come from the matter of the fruit flesh and which are by nature destined for the growth of new life.

With this I have arrived at the most important point of the question of nutrition, in which some vegetarians are more backward than the cultured eaters. The essential, actually power-bringing of all food is the aroma, and from this point of view everything cooked is almost worthless and only ballast. As long as this ballast is mastered and excreted again, and the decomposed substances are not yet attacked, man with cooked food actually lives on less than the fruit eater. And for this reason Dr. Dewen is right when he claims that thousands of people starve to death by eating all day long. From this new point of view, the series of foods is called: air, light, water, fragrances, especially those of flowers, aromatic and nutritious fruit not diluted by cultivation. St. Catherine is said to have lived for more than 10 years in fresh health in a rose garden with water and the host, and Professor Jäger speaks in all seriousness of a "scent therapy". Now it becomes clearer and more understandable why the human being, filled with rotting and fermenting substances inside, becomes weak already after one day of fasting. Not only the blood-poisoning substances paralyze and tire the motor and sensitive nerves, but this and especially the poisonous gases which are formed by their dissolution in the blood when the food supply ceases. Now it becomes understandable why the Indian fakir endures the fasting the longest - he lives essentially on dates, and why I survived the fasting the easiest, having previously lived essentially on cherries. An ideally healthy person would have to get tired and hungry much later, precisely because he does not or almost does not "metabolize" as the cultured man does. "Dormir c'est manger" (to sleep is to eat) wants to say that sleep is more important than eating. A dog can last 60-70 days without food, but not 10 days without sleep. No one will claim that he would become stronger by eating continuously, while one can be freed from heavy fatigue in short, quiet sleep. The art of sleeping is much more important than eating, especially during illness.

With these explanations, but especially with my fasting tests, the theory of nutrition has not been shaken anew with regard to the amount of food to be ingested, but I believe that I have opened a breach in the scientific concepts of the metabolism of man. Thus, new points of view for the application of purely natural dietetics, as well as nutritional therapy, which is also the only strictly natural way of healing, could be established, through which man can attain paradisiacal health and unimagined pleasures. I have lingered a little long on the physiological side of my theses, because it seems to me to be very important.

I have to show now in the further that also the "spiritual evils" of mankind originate from the same source as the bodily diseases. Rather it would have to be proved that the first-mentioned and all other degenerative phenomena listed in my thesis are to be derived from the disease and thus from overeating and wrong food. For the disease itself, as well as for all its sequelae, there are still some other causes and circumstances to accuse. I know this very well. Up to now, however, the latter have been the minor ones, always so much emphasized over the importance of the stomach in the "forge of destiny". ("Man is what he eats," Feuerbach). Strictly speaking, one cannot prove anything by words. Only facts are conclusive, and he who has accomplished facts may demand faith in them. Even the exact science of the scholars, apart from the facts of experience just only indirect knowledge, i.e. faith, only with the difference that the "authorities" concerned must not be pope, but at least professor or doctor, in order to be considered "infallible". One sees, the system is always the same; only the names, persons and power holders change. Woe to him who dares to doubt the dogmas of the scholars! He is "burned", as in former times, but spiritually i.e. hushed up.

From my experiments and my conception of disease it is clear that there is no such thing as a perfectly healthy human being. What the today's nervous and brain pathology calls mental diseases, for that also my view applies in so far as I have already mentioned that the meat consumption produces alcohol craving and is therefore also cause of alcoholism and most mental diseases, while one will never see that a vegetarian perishes from alcohol. It is well known that often people became mentally ill and even insane during involuntary fasts, for example during the siege of Paris. As an experimenter I have to state here again that this pathological influence on mind and spirit only becomes strongly apparent if before the f̲a̲s̲t̲i̲n̲g̲,̲ ̲m̲u̲c̲h̲ ̲m̲e̲a̲t̲ ̲w̲a̲s̲ ̲e̲a̲t̲e̲n̲,̲ ̲i̲f̲ ̲t̲h̲u̲s̲ ̲i̲n̲ ̲t̲h̲e̲ ̲b̲l̲o̲o̲d̲ ̲a̲n̲d̲ b̲r̲a̲i̲n̲ ̲c̲i̲r̲c̲l̲i̲n̲g̲ ̲c̲o̲r̲p̲s̲e̲ ̲p̲o̲i̲s̲o̲n̲s̲ ̲o̲f̲ ̲b̲a̲c̲k̲w̲a̲r̲d̲ ̲f̲o̲o̲d̲ ̲r̲e̲m̲a̲i̲n̲d̲e̲r̲s̲ ̲a̲r̲e̲ ̲t̲h̲e̲ c̲a̲u̲s̲e̲.̲ In the scientific view of eating one's own flesh during fasting, which is also held by Dr. Kellogg, it must be considered that 70-80 percent of the flesh consists of water, and that according to my earlier explanations probably only the diseased cells of one's own flesh are attacked, which is already evident from the fact that the more perfect one's health is, the less weight is lost when abstaining from food (fakirs). With the extreme of psychopathic phenomena (alcoholism and autointoxication by own corpse poisons), however, also the influence, even if only indirectly, is proved, which wrong food intake and overfeeding exert on the spirit. But what is truth as extreme, that is true also in the small. Thus a correct thinking, an "immaculate" cognition, the pure reason of man, is questioned the moment the first traces of decomposed cellular or food material or of stimulants (poisons) circulate in the blood and in the brain. Philosophizing, all brooding and questioning, science itself, and especially medical science, if there is such a thing at all (healing was, is and will always remain an art), would have to be regarded as pathological phenomena. Even if necessary for today's mankind, they are basically harmful to health physically and also spiritually, and that is the decisive thing. All so-called "progress" of today is in the last analysis in the service of decline. Nietzsche himself calls all philosophy decadence and the vaunted Kant the greatest cripple of intellect of his century. Maumner writes two volumes to prove that language has brought Babylonian confusion, that no one understands the books that fill our libraries, and that all questions of existence are answered with as many yeses as noes.

Who is informed about the newest researches and spiritual currents, knows that all still so seemingly fixed knowledge has come to shake, even the natural science. Many scholars, even modern ones, have come to the conclusion that we can know nothing and will know nothing (ignorabimus). And I say that we do not need to know anything. Well, mankind needs it for its alleged progress, but man does not need it. For what then science, if everything again comes down to error and harmfulness and thinking is pathological in itself, as long as (man is not completely healthy!).

Thinking means: to compare facts, observations; to connect logically. All world views and sciences suffer from the fact that they do not look at the world, i.e. not artistically as "sensual manifestation" but to tear down everything, also the organisms, and to look at them through the microscope. I still come to speak about the "supersensible revelation" as only healthy and useful thoughts of man. Even the Häkean "world riddle", what the prehistoric man was, I solve by the experiment. Give me a group of mentally and physically degenerated people. I want to make them healthy in the forest, to speak with Rousseau, by fasting and fruit diet. It will then be shown whether they sink without the "blessing" of the culture to the semi-monkey, or whether they do not put all "present" in beauty, strength and intelligence in the shade.

When man deviated from the only correct food with the Fall, the whole misery of his existence began; this is written exactly in the Bible. With the intake of wrong and surplus food also the self-purification process begins, i.e. the disease process, which is kept in check, i.e. latent, only by increasing the amount of food, by stimulants and later by allopathic means. With regard to causes of disease there is great confusion and profoundest ignorance today. But with regard to all spiritual questions of existence, and especially about the causes of "evil", "evil", etc., our time surpasses all others in confusion, contradiction and opposition, as I have already shown above. And nevertheless there can be only one truth and only one answer to all why, why and wherefrom. Culture and with it property was necessary only when man ate too much and wrongly, and the first who fenced a piece of land was not the first sacrilegious man (Rousseau), but that was the first culture man. He did this to protect himself and his numerous children from hunger, which he had begotten as a result of the sexual drive increased by wrong food. Thereby his food became "mixed", and likewise mixed became his "thinking", his character. He became "refined", i.e. he invented means to cover his nakedness, and to deceive his neighbors, who were perhaps still naked, namely in the choice of sex, since his beauty had also suffered as a result of the wrong food. Thus the clothing industry was born - a finger branch for the friends of the naked. About the connection of beauty and food still gives the experiment today.

With property, freedom, equality and fraternity came to an end at the same time. The more one owns, the more one is "possessed". The inequality of the people does not come, as Rousseau means, from the inequality of the property, but from the inequality of the nutrition. But this can be equal only with the biologically correct one, and that is fruit diet.

So with the wrong food the social question was born, and this then therefore never, at least not in the sense of socialism or anarchism, will be solved, because just the future state has the equality of the people, not only in relation to the right, but namely in relation to their properties, as a prerequisite. That s precisely the vegetarians are so different in their views and so quarrelsome, does not refute my assertion; for precisely among them there are the most gradations in nutrition. But an industrial people will not feed on fruit. This is the real reason for the utopia of the "future state" - a finger pointing for social enthusiasts.

With the further increase of the food supply the discovery of stimulants became conditional of spices, tobacco, coffee, alcohol etc., in order to stimulate the body weakened under the load of the overnutrition and to make it "afloat" — a finger pointer for one-sided abstinence hawks. The now particularly strong sex drive produced the first "people", and with this multiplication the brotherhood in the natural and in the ethical sense went more and more into the break. Thus, however, a dictator became necessary, and the most beautiful, strongest, noblest and cleverest rose to this position. This was the one who had deviated least from the law of natural nourishment, in whose veins still rolled noble, i.e. pure blood. With it the first ruler appeared, and with it also slaves and servitude, the "God's nobility", the first state. But also the blood of the prince degenerated for designated reasons and with it his ruling power sank. Another competes with him. The people separates, peoples, states arise and with it the war from quarrel about land and property for food purposes. Now a social and moral bait becomes necessary, and the winner in the war is just as well called "bad" as the stronger in the fight for existence — a finger pointer for moralists, peace hawks and Nietzsche opponents. The people grows to the nation and industry becomes necessary to increase the food and the traffic, while until now the "cursed" field had done the mischief alone. Now the food and stimulants and with it the regulation of the sex drive are "refined". Prostitution arises — a finger pointer for "morality apostles".

A thousand times more "hunger for love" remains unsatisfied than need for food. Instead, more is eaten and drunk. In the proverb that one could live on air and love, there is a large spark of truth.

Now more and more must be cooked, fried, baked, and so much food must be fabricated that three quarters of all mankind and the female sex have become slaves to this work. On the other hand, I have calculated, on the basis of long experiments, that ten real full-grown fruit trees in the Central European climate can permanently feed a family of four with very few ingredients. One sees: the "paradise" is still to be had; one needs it only to want.

Agriculture is physiologically a nonsense, because apart from unnecessary stimulants, to which I also count meat, it essentially produces carbohydrates, which the organism must first convert into glucose, which one can have in the fruits directly, effortlessly and without the "sweat of his face" (Mos. 3,17 and 18). Besides, it is just the carbohydrates (starch-flour food) whose residues form pathological foci in the intestinal mucus and stomach - a finger pointer for bread and porridge vegetarians and national economists!

Dr. Weiniger, whose book "Sex and Character" has caused such a sensation as seldom another, proves that there is only one kind of genius, namely the universal genius, and that is the founder of religion. These have all fasted in order thereby to arrive at the "revelation of a divine wisdom." In modern terms and reasonably interpreted, this means: they exposed themselves in pure mountain or desert air to the voluntary, deliberately induced disease process by withholding food until the last pathologically developed cell was eliminated in the sense of my opinion. Only in this state a completely pure brain activity occurs and a receiving of valuable thoughts, as it were an instinctive, will-less self-generating of the highest all-knowledge, which the poets of strong times called "inspiration".

This is "supersensible revelation" in the natural sense, physiology of the healthy thinking of the universal genius and founder of religion who, according to Dr. Weiniger, knows everything worth knowing without having learned it. With these abilities, however, physical and mental qualities of higher degree enter at the same time. I will speak about this more precisely and in more detail in another place, and I will discuss in more detail my occult abilities which I have already achieved, even if still to a modest extent. This is only a hint for miracle believers and also for the all denying "enlightened" and "moderns". I will discuss the transcendental question on another occasion, since it does not belong here, although it too can only come down to a biological and therefore basically diegetic problem, as absurd as this seems to be. At least this question is not dismissed with the modern phrase of the "dark nothing", which actually expresses only a wish that it may be so, because one is not sure of his thing in spite of all so-called enlightenment and goes over it with a "non tangere".

With this I believe to have done justice to my previous assertions as far as space allows, that here is the source for the solution of the highest and most valuable questions of existence is undisputed. As a modern representative of asceticism I differ essentially from those of all millennia.

I have recognized that asceticism (fasting) is not an end in itself and, if thoroughly carried out, is necessary only once, whereby alone one becomes physically and spiritually completely healthy and thus comes only to correct, also sensual pleasures, of which today's mankind has no more idea. I further differ from other representatives of this direction in that I do not want to convert the world, mankind, because this is a clear impossibility for me. Here a new world opens only for few. I have already arrived at the gate of it and will try, as far as it is in my powers, to go further, because I recognize in this direction the goal set for man by the law of nature. Whoever wants to go with me towards this goal of unconditional, mystery-free and above all disease-free existence, I welcome him, and if he does not yet "believe", then I simply invite him into the school of the attempt and he will experience that the most unbelievable becomes natural to him.